The Good Gut Anti-Inflammatory Diet

Beat Whole Body Inflammation And Live Longer, Happier, Healthier And Younger

Prof Phil Hansbro

16pt

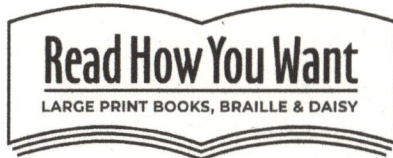

Read How You Want
LARGE PRINT BOOKS, BRAILLE & DAISY

Copyright Page from the Original Book

TABLE OF CONTENTS

Foreword   i

Introduction   vi

    1: Inflammation overload – what it looks like, and why it matters   1

    2: How does chronic inflammation cause disease?   22

    3: Ageing and inflammation: inflammageing   33

    4: Welcome to the microbiome   41

    5: How our gut microbiome influences inflammation   54

    6: How diet shapes our microbiome   68

    7: The rise of the modern Western diet   90

    8: Minimising inflammation: lifestyle and microbiome approaches   115

    9: What to eat – and why   128

    10: Meal planner   158

BREAKFAST   162

    MANGO & VANILLA YOGHURT POTS WITH PISTACHIO & MINT
    TOPPER   162

    BROWN RICE & BUCKWHEAT PORRIDGE WITH ROASTED
    STRAWBERRIES & MIXED SEED SPRINKLE   164

    BASIL-FRIED EGGS WITH RADICCHIO & ALMOND TOAST   166

    SIMPLE SHAKSHUKA   168

    SPICED AVOCADO TOAST WITH ARTICHOKE-CAPSICUM
    SALSA   170

    WHOLEMEAL BANANA & NUTMEG BREAKFAST MUFFINS   172

    STRAWBERRY PUDDINGS WITH STRAWBERRY & DRAGONFRUIT
    SALAD   174

    OVERNIGHT OATS WITH PAPAYA & KIWIFRUIT   176

    RYE & KEFIR HOTCAKES WITH LEMONY BERRIES   178

    COCONUT & TAHINI BREAKFAST PORRIDGE WITH SPICED
    BANANA   180

    HERB OMELETTES WITH FRIED TOMATOES   182

    GREEN GODDESS BREAKFAST SMOOTHIE WITH GOAT'S MILK
    YOGHURT   184

    GREEN EGGS, NO HAM   186

    FRITTATA WITH SAUTÉED GREENS, SWEET POTATO &
    BROCCOLI   188

LUNCH   190

    CABBAGE ROLLS WITH KALE, OAT & PARMESAN FILLING   190

    ROAST CHICKEN, SAUERKRAUT & PROVOLONE PAN
    BAGNAT   192

    SOY & ORANGE GLAZED TEMPEH WITH ZOODLE SALAD   194

    CHICKEN PAD THAI   196

    MUSSEL & MIXED BEAN HOTPOT   198

    SIMPLE SUSHI WITH PRAWNS, AVOCADO & SEAWEED   200

    SARDINE BOQUERONES WITH GRILLED SOURDOUGH FINGERS
    & ROASTED CABBAGE SALAD   202

    HOT SMOKED TROUT, PUMPKIN & FENNEL SALAD PLATE WITH
    TURMERIC & CITRUS DRESSING   204

    SEARED SCALLOPS WITH CARROT PURÉE & HERBS   206

    PRAWN, SHALLOT & SNOW PEA RICE PAPER ROLLS   208

    PARSLEY, DILL & BROAD BEAN FALAFELS WITH MINT-GARLIC
    YOGHURT   210

    CHICKEN SATAY SKEWERS   212

    SPINACH & BROCCOLINI CREPES   214

    GREEN LINGUINE WITH RICOTTA, LEMON & BREADCRUMBS 216

DINNER   218

    GRASS-FED LAMB LOIN CHOPS WITH WHOLE-WHEAT KIMCHI
    DUMPLINGS IN PEA & GARLIC HASH   218

    RAINBOW TROUT 'AL CARTOCCIO' WITH KIMCHI,
    BROCCOLINI, HEART OF PALM & CITRUS SALSA   220

    LINGUINE 'AGLIO E OLIO'   222

    PRAWN & ONION KEBABS WITH GRILLED CORN & BEAN
    SALAD   224

    BAHARAT KOFTE WITH GOLDEN ROASTED BRUSSELS
    SPROUTS   226

    SLOW-COOKED LAMB SHOULDER   228

    ROASTED MUSHROOM RISOTTO   230

    CICERI E TRIA: PUGLIESE PASTA & CHICKPEAS   232

    VEGETARIAN MASSAMAN CURRY OF POTATOES, CELERY &
    TOFU   234

    ROASTED MACKEREL IN GREEN HERB CRUST   236

FLORENTINE-STYLE BARBECUED T-BONE WITH HERB BUTTER 238

BRAISED & CHARGRILLED OCTOPUS WITH GARDEN CRUDITÉS 240

GRILLED CHICKEN & TOMATO WHITE CORN TOSTADAS 242

KOREAN-STYLE BRAISED BEEF SHORT RIBS 244

DESSERTS & SNACKS 246

SUGAR-FREE RYE & BERRY SHORTCAKES WITH YOGHURT 246

SIMPLE VANILLA-LEMON-RICOTTA CHEESECAKE WITH CHERRY COMPOTE 248

MIXED MELON SALAD WITH LIME & MARJORAM 250

EASY OLIVE OIL CHOCOLATE-CHUNK COOKIES 252

DATE, MACADAMIA & CINNAMON ROLLS 254

HOMEMADE CHEESE STICKS 256

WHIPPED VANILLA CUSTARD WITH APRICOTS & CRISP PARMESAN-WALNUT WAFERS 258

MOCHA CAKE WITH CAROB SYRUP & GRAPE SALAD 260

DANISH BUTTER BISCUITS 262

CAFFÈ CORRETTO PANNA COTTA WITH TWICE-COOKED BERRIES 264

BROWN BUTTER & RASPBERRY CAKE 266

EASY LEMON TEA CAKE 268

SUGAR-FREE CROSTOLI 270

PEACH & ALMOND TART 272

Dr Clare Bailey's: BONUS DAY OF RECIPES 274

SCRAMBLED EGGS ON SOURDOUGH TOAST WITH SMOKED SALMON & HOMEMADE SAUERKRAUT 275

EASY MISO SOUP WITH PRAWNS & NOODLES (ADAPTED FROM THE FAST 800 EASY) 277

EASY MOROCCAN CHICKEN TAGINE 279

CHEESY PARMESAN BISCUITS WITH ROSEMARY 282

About the author 285

Contributors 287

Endnotes 289

References 315

Back Cover Material   361
Index   363

Foreword

Dr Michael Mosley

I am delighted to have this chance to write a foreword to *The Good Gut Anti-Inflammatory Diet,* as inflammation and the gut are subjects I have a particular interest in. I am also a long-term fan of the work of Professor Mathew Vadas and the Centenary Institute, where he is Executive Director. The Centenary Institute is a world-leading independent medical research organisation that does groundbreaking work with a special focus on cancer, inflammation and heart disease. As you will discover when you read this book, these areas of health are intimately linked and closely tied into gut health.

I first got interested in the gut and the mysterious microbes that live down in the murky depths of our intestines when I made a TV documentary called *Ulcer Wars* for the BBC and the ABC, way back in 1994. As the title suggests, the program was about gastric ulcers, which were once very common in the Western world and widely believed to be triggered by stress and a poor diet. Gastric ulcers were seen as an incurable condition that was best treated by taking medication that could reduce levels of acid in the stomach.

But as the documentary revealed, in Perth, Western Australia, there were a couple of doctors, Robin Warren and Barry Marshall, who were convinced that existing theories about the causes of gastric ulcers were wrong and that most gastric ulcers happen as the result of a gut infection by a previously unknown bacterium that they had identified and named *Helicobacter pylori* (*H. pylori*). They believed that one of the main reasons gastric ulcers occur is because the body responds to infection by producing more stomach acid, which fails to kill the bugs, but which can cause ulcers.

Their theory was largely dismissed by the scientific community, so Dr Marshall decided to take matters into his own hands and attempt a bold, eye-catching experiment. He asked a technician to brew up a flask of *H. pylori*, which he then swallowed. 'It didn't taste good,' Barry told me. 'Like swamp water.'

A few days later, feeling seriously ill, Dr Marshall had himself endoscoped; a small tube was passed down his throat and into his stomach. Samples of his now inflamed stomach lining were biopsied, and these revealed that his gut had indeed been colonised by *H. pylori*. Barry took a course of antibiotics, which he had previously shown could kill *H. pylori*, and soon his stomach was back to normal.

When the documentary was first broadcast in 1994 it got a hostile reaction from some parts of the medical community, while others sat up and paid notice. Over time views changed, and I'm delighted to be able to report that in 2005,

11 years after this brave self-experiment, Marshall and Warren won the Nobel Prize for Medicine for their work, which completely transformed the way that gastric ulcers are treated, and improved the lives of millions.

Their work also inspired a new generation of scientists who, in the 1990s, began seriously exploring the wonderful world of the microbiome, the 2–3 kilos of microbes that live in your gut and play such a critical role in our health.

The microbiome explorers were helped by the development of cheap and sensitive technology which meant it became possible to detect fragments of DNA and RNA in samples of people's faeces, and from that infer the sort of microbes that must be living in that person's gut. I have had my faeces sampled on a couple of occasions and found the results revealing.

But it wasn't until 2012, when I discovered that I had type 2 diabetes, that my interest in diet, and the impact that what you eat (or don't eat) has on your microbiome and metabolic health, really took off. Again the turning point was making a documentary for the BBC, this time called *Eat, Fast, Live Longer.*

In the course of making that documentary I came across research on the benefits of intermittent fasting and put myself on what I called a 5:2 diet, eating around a quarter of my normal calories two days a week. I also gave up sugary snacks and switched to eating a healthy

Mediterranean-style diet, rich in vegetables, olive oil, oily fish and nuts.

Thanks to a combination of intermittent fasting and a healthier diet, I lost nine kilograms in eight weeks and 10 centimetres around my waist. Even better, my blood sugars returned to normal, where they have stayed ever since. And, interestingly enough, my gut microbiome also improved, with a marked increase in something called the Simpson index, which is a mark of microbe diversity.

Since then there have been multiple studies which have shown that switching from a typical Australian diet to a Mediterranean diet has multiple benefits, not only for your body but also for your brain. The SMILEs Study, published by researchers from the Food and Mood Centre at Deakin University in Victoria in 2017, was one of the first to show that a change in diet can have a profound beneficial effect on people with moderate to severe depression.[1]

And as for intermittent fasting and the gut, studies by the Erasmus University Medical Center in the Netherlands, among others, have shown that intermittent fasting boosts levels of 'good' bacteria, like *Lachnospiraceae*, which in turn make a short-chain fatty acid called butyrate, which sends anti-inflammatory signals to the immune system.[2] You'll be reading more about butyrate later in the book.

This is a hugely interesting area of research, and I hope I have whetted your appetite for what is to come.

Introduction

Professor Mathew Vadas AO MB BS FRACP FRCPA PhD DSc FAHMS Executive Director, Centenary Institute

The Centenary Institute is a world-leading research organisation working on the most complex health challenges of cancer, inflammation and cardiovascular disease. It was formed under an Act of the New South Wales Parliament to mark the 100th anniversary of the dual foundation of Royal Prince Alfred Hospital and the Faculty of Medicine at the University of Sydney.

Scientists here at the Centenary Institute and around the world work tirelessly to better understand the causes of – and therefore potential treatments for – the diseases that continue to affect our lives and the lives of those we love. Enormous gains have been made: breakthroughs in medical research have led to our lifespans doubling in the last 100 years, and we've made significant leaps in our understanding of the biology and mechanisms of disease. Thanks to this work, we now understand many ways to address the problem of disease, including lifestyle changes, new or repurposed drugs, and biological therapies.

But this book is about one particular area of study that has been a major focus of the Centenary Institute: inflammation. While it may seem mundane at first, we believe that understanding inflammation is the key to unlocking a new era of treatments and cures for many of the deadliest and most prominent diseases affecting humanity today.

Inflammation is fundamental to the way that our body's immune system reacts to injury and is critical in resolving infection or trauma. However, it also forms the foundation of many prevalent acute and chronic conditions. Chronic smouldering inflammation – moderate inflammation that lasts a significant period of time – leads to shorter lifespans and lower quality of life, as well as contributing to some forms of dementia, lung diseases, allergies, autoimmune diseases, and the progression of cancer and cardiovascular disease.

Happily, even in the face of such a list, there are things that we know:
First, gut health can affect chronic inflammation – both for good and for bad.

Second, we can affect our gut health through our diet and the foods we eat.

Third, scientists are learning more about gut health and how to harness it every day.

At the forefront of this research is one of the world's leading inflammation researchers, Professor Philip Hansbro, Director of the Centenary UTS Centre for Inflammation, Australia's first research organisation dedicated exclusively to studying the mechanisms underlying inflammation.

Professor Hansbro and his team have more than 25 years' experience exploring how the immune system, and in particular inflammation, contributes to the progression of chronic respiratory diseases. Professor Hansbro has come to the realisation that inflammation can be managed. While we can use drugs when things have seriously gone wrong, a healthy lifestyle, including attention to our diet, can help prevent diseases before they take hold. Therefore, it's important for everyone to understand some of the ways inflammation arises and where it can be controlled.

This book delivers practical information about how inflammation works in your body, and gives a lifelong framework that will provide you with tools to limit inflammation now, and when facing challenges in the future. In closing, please enjoy *The Good Gut Anti-Inflammatory Diet* and the knowledge within its pages, from the charts and illustrations, the nutrition and lifestyle advice, and especially the delicious recipes from Ed Halmagyi and Dr Clare Bailey. I hope it helps you lead a happier, healthier, and younger life.

Inflammation overload – what it looks like, and why it matters

For the first time in global history, our life expectancy is getting shorter the wealthier we get. Despite major advances in healthcare, modernisation – the move away from an agricultural-based society to an industrial one – came with an epidemic of chronic diseases.

We now know that inflammatory processes in the body are behind many common and serious diseases – a very long, and surprisingly varied, list that includes infectious diseases like pneumonia, influenza and COVID-19, as well as chronic diseases like asthma, chronic obstructive pulmonary disease (COPD), arthritis, heart/cardiovascular disease, inflammatory bowel diseases, neurological disease, kidney disease and liver disease. We suspect many cancers also have an inflammatory component.

Most of these diseases aren't single-organ diseases affecting just one part of the body. It might be hard to visualise, but these diseases actually involve an underlying state of whole-body inflammation (that is, involving many of our bodily systems – also known as 'systemic' inflammation).

The health burden associated with the modern upsurge in inflammatory diseases, both for individual sufferers themselves and for public health systems all over the world, is staggering. It really isn't an exaggeration to say we're living in an inflammation pandemic.

But what's causing this modern health disaster? What does it have to do with our gastrointestinal system and gut bacteria? What *is* inflammation, and what can we do about it?

Good inflammation: our guardian angel

'Good' inflammation is our immune system's natural defence against harmful microbes, irritants, chemicals and toxins. Good inflammation keeps us alive and is essential for healing us when we're injured. It's short-acting and purposeful – a specific and appropriate response to natural stimuli (e.g. healing a cut or fighting off a cold or other infection).

Chronic inflammation: snapshot of a silent killer

You can think of 'bad' inflammation as the fundamental cause of most disease: a lot of common, serious diseases are driven by inflammatory processes in the body. Bad inflammation happens when the body over-reacts to stimuli in the modern world, or when our immune system is over-activated for a long time. Inflammation overload can affect all our organs and damage our health – or worse, even kill us.

Inflammation breakthrough!

By reducing inflammation in our bodies, we can help prevent and treat disease.

Respiratory diseases

Respiratory diseases are the most common cause of poor health and death worldwide. Like most inflammatory conditions, respiratory diseases can be both acute (short-term) and chronic (long-term or constantly recurring).

The common cold, pneumonia, influenza and COVID-19 are all acute respiratory diseases, although some might have long-term effects (like long COVID). Like other conditions caused by an infection, they're a result of excessive inflammation brought on by the immune system working overtime to clear the infection. Asthma, COPD and tuberculosis are more chronic.

People who already have high levels of underlying inflammation in their body are more likely to develop respiratory diseases. Once they develop a chronic respiratory disease, they can also experience short-term, quick flare-ups in symptoms ('exacerbations' or 'attacks') – like an asthma attack, for example.

Let's look at some of these diseases in more detail.

Asthma

Asthma is an allergic disease of the airways. People with asthma are more sensitive to infection, smoke, and other stimuli that don't affect other people. Some asthma is linked to acute viral infections that cause inflammation when we're very young (0–2 years old) and get worse when we develop allergies to things like dust, smoke, infection, house dust mites and pollen (which is especially noteworthy, given that global warming means pollen seasons last longer).

Being exposed to these allergens and other stimuli inflames and tightens the airways, leading to the wheezing and difficulty breathing typical of an asthma attack.

Asthma affects over 330 million people around the world. In Europe and the US,[3] it costs about $1900–$3100 per person every year; in Australia, the yearly cost is $28 billion.

Emphysema (COPD)

Emphysema is a main feature of chronic obstructive pulmonary disease (COPD), which also involves chronic bronchitis (chronic inflammation of the airways). It's caused by smoking and long-term exposure to air pollution, both indoor (e.g. cooking smoke) and outdoor (e.g. environmental smoke such as from diesel or petrol fumes, brushfire, and infection). Emphysema is the third most common cause of death globally.[4]

Low-grade inflammation happens every time we're exposed to cigarettes, air pollution and other challenges. Although it goes away easily, repeated or constant exposure overwhelms our lungs' ability to repair itself, causing irreparable damage to the airways and gas exchange cells (alveoli). This leads to severe breathing difficulties and eventually death.

COPD is becoming more common as the global population ages, air pollution levels soar, forests burn due to land clearing for farming, and bushfires related to global warming become more frequent. Over 50% of people with COPD have never smoked.

COPD affects about 300 million people worldwide. For a group of 28 European countries, the combined cost of COPD is €48.4 billion.[5] About 20% of people die from COPD-related issues, like heart disease and stroke.

At a glance

Disease	Cause	Numbers
Common cold	Mostly rhinoviruses, some coronaviruses and other viruses	People get two to three colds each year on average, costing the global economy about $25 billion a year.[6]
COVID-19	Severe Acute Respiratory Syndrome Coronavirus-2 (SARS-CoV-2)	In the first year of the pandemic, 1.9 million people died. The global costs have been astronomical. Roughly two years into the pandemic, the International Monetary Fund estimated that $28 trillion was lost in revenue alone.
Flu (influenza)	Influenza A virus	About 250,000–500,000 people die every year from seasonal influenza. The virus can also cause pandemics. Spanish influenza killed 20–40 million people in 1918–19: that's more deaths than the whole First World War.
Pneumonia	*Streptococcus pneumoniae, Haemophilus influenzae* and other bacteria, and some viruses	Kills about 2.5 million people each year, mostly children and older adults.[7] It's estimated to cost Europe €10.1 billion a year, and the US $17 billion a year.
Tuberculosis	*Mycobacterium tuberculosis*	Causes 1.4 million deaths every year, costing about $15 billion in prevention, treatment and research.[8]

Allergic conditions

People who have eczema, hives, hay fever, sinusitis, asthma or a food or drug allergy tend to have multiple allergic conditions, since the same underlying inflammatory process affects different tissues in different ways. In fact, allergies often develop in a sequence known as the atopic (or allergic) march.[9]

Breathing in or swallowing the offending allergen releases defensive chemicals (e.g. histamine), setting off symptoms ranging in severity from mildly irritating to life threatening.

About half of school-aged children have an allergy of some kind.[10] Over 170 different foods can cause allergic reactions; 2.7% of kids have peanut allergies. Interestingly, people raised with pets – particularly dogs or farm animals – seem to be protected from developing allergies.[11] Food allergies cost individuals about $8000 per year,[12] while hay fever costs about $5 billion globally every year.[13]

Atopic march

The progression of allergic diseases from infancy to adulthood. For example, you might get hives as a baby, which progress to a peanut allergy when you're a toddler, then develops into asthma when you hit school age.

Inflammatory bowel diseases

Inflammatory conditions of the gut, like Crohn's disease and ulcerative colitis,[14] have become far more common over the past few decades. Crohn's disease causes deep inflammation in the gut wall (usually at the end of the small intestine). It's associated with smoking – the inflammation is similar to lung inflammation in smokers. Ulcerative colitis causes ulcers and a chronic surface inflammation of the gut wall (colon/large intestine) and has more of an allergic component.

Collectively known as inflammatory bowel diseases (IBDs), these conditions have serious symptoms: diarrhoea and urgent bowel movements, stomach pain, rectal bleeding from ulcers and weight loss, to name a few. IBDs now affect almost seven million people globally.[15] The lifetime cost of having an IBD is about $400,000–$600,000.[16]

Autoimmune conditions

Inflammation is the underlying factor in over 100 autoimmune diseases,[17] which affect about 50 million Americans and cost over $100 billion per year.[18]

In autoimmune diseases, our bodies see our own healthy cells and tissues as foreign invaders and try to remove them. Autoimmunity also plays a part in COPD (see section entitled "Emphysema (COPD)") and inflammatory bowel diseases (see section entitled "Respiratory diseases").

At a glance

Disease	Cause	Symptoms include:
Arthritis	Our body's immune cells (B cells) produce antibodies that attach themselves to the surface of joints. They cause inflammatory responses that destroy the joints' surfaces.	Joint pain Swelling Stiffness and erosion

Disease	Cause	Symptoms include:
Lupus (systemic lupus erythematosus)	Antibodies attach themselves to different tissues. They cause inflammation and damage the respiratory tract and joints along with blood cells, nerves and kidneys.	Aching and swollen joints Fever Fatigue Chest pain/pleurisy Hair loss Seizures Light sensitivity
Multiple sclerosis (MS)	Inflammation and parts of the immune system attack, and eventually destroy, nerve cells (which weakens muscle function). Infections are likely to be the initial driver.	Pain Muscle weakness and spasms Impaired coordination Blindness
Psoriasis	Inflammatory responses make skin cells reproduce too quickly, causing a build-up of T cells in our skin.	Dry, itchy, raised skin patches with silvery-white flakes (called scales).
Type 1 diabetes (diabetes mellitus)	Inflammation and the immune system damage the beta cells that produce insulin in the pancreas, making it harder for our bodies to metabolise glucose.	Mainly frequent urination, thirst and hunger. Other symptoms include unexplained weight loss, upset stomach, vomiting, fatigue, and frequent skin or genital tract infections.
Vasculitis/angiitis/arteritis	Inflammation and the immune system damages blood vessels, enlarging them and making them leaky or likely to collapse anywhere in the body. It can affect several organs at the same time (e.g. skin, brain, eyes). It's linked to allergic responses, arthritis and lupus.	Relatively mild fever Appetite and weight loss Fatigue and skin rashes More severe outcomes include stroke, heart attack and kidney disease.

Other, rarer, autoimmune conditions include Guillain-Barré syndrome, chronic inflammatory demyelinating polyneuropathy, Graves' disease, thyroiditis and myasthenia gravis.

Heart disease

Inflammation is common in heart disease, though research into the role inflammation plays in heart attacks is ongoing. Major risk factors include smoking and smoke exposure, high blood pressure and high blood cholesterol. These risk factors lead to fats (called plaques) being deposited in blood vessels, thickening or hardening the arteries, which induces inflammatory responses. It can also lead to a heart attack if the plaques rupture and form blood clots.

Cardiovascular disease is the single most common cause of illness and death. By 2030, the global cost of heart disease is estimated to reach $1.04 trillion.

Neurological conditions

Inflammation is also common in neurological conditions, for example stroke, Alzheimer's disease, Parkinson's disease, Huntington's disease and traumatic brain injury.

Neurological conditions have gone up almost 30% in the last two decades.[19] They cause nine million deaths a year, mainly from stroke, Alzheimer's disease, other forms of dementia, and meningitis. In Australia, brain disorders cost $74 billion a year, and $800 billion in the US.[20]

Stroke

Inflammation can play an important role in stroke. Inflammatory cells, and the chemical signals they release, build up in the walls of blood vessels; this build-up becomes systemic, meaning it happens throughout our body. Eventually, the plaque ruptures and forms blood clots that stop blood flow to the brain. Stroke can result in severe brain damage and death.[21] Symptoms include sudden weakness in the arm and/or leg on one side of the body, weakness in the face (with drooping), speaking difficulties, loss of vision, trouble walking and severe headache.

Alzheimer's disease

We now think brain inflammation is important in Alzheimer's disease, which is characterised by the build-up of a molecule called beta-amyloid in the brain. We don't yet know what causes it. At normal levels, beta-amyloid has antimicrobial and antiviral effects, and is brought on by inflammatory responses, suggesting a link between beta-amyloid levels, infections and inflammation.[22] Beta-amyloid (and the inflammatory responses involved) also increases with ageing. Symptoms include memory loss, mood changes, confusion, disorientation and difficulty problem-solving or finding the right words.

Parkinson's disease

Parkinson's disease involves losing a specific type of brain neuron that controls body movement. Infection and inflammation are increasingly linked to the destruction of these cells.

When we study the brains of Parkinson's disease patients, we see antibodies present against these neurons, as well as elevated levels of inflammatory cells and their chemical signals.[23] Symptoms include speech and writing difficulties, uncontrollable tremors and slow movement, with rigid muscles, stooped posture and balance issues.

Huntington's disease

Changes in the huntingtin protein in the brain, as well as different organs and tissues, lead to Huntington's disease. We think peripheral inflammation precedes symptoms of the disease.[24] Symptoms involve muscle and functional impairment, cognitive decline and psychiatric issues.

Traumatic brain injury

High-impact blows to the head and injuries from car crashes or other head traumas can lead to brain injury, with significant physical impairments that last weeks, months or years after the injury.[25] These ongoing issues are related to inflammation in the brain, which also causes swelling. The inflammation is similar to inflammation in multiple sclerosis and Alzheimer's disease.

Brain injuries are the most common cause of disability and death in children and young adults. Symptoms include cognitive impairment, dementia, muscle dysfunction and psychiatric issues.

Meningitis

Meningitis has many forms, and all are bacterial or viral infectious diseases. The bacteria that usually cause these diseases are part of the normal bacteria that happily live in our throat – in fact, at any one time, 10% of us have these bacteria. But when they make it into our bloodstream, these same bacteria trigger inflammatory responses that circulate to the brain and cause meningitis, a serious (and potentially fatal) that requires immediate medical attention. Symptoms include very sudden high fever, severe headache, stiff neck and light sensitivity.

Reproductive tract conditions

Inflammation from infections can affect our reproductive tracts. This includes pelvic inflammatory disease, tubal infertility, prostatitis, epididymitis and orchitis, among other things. Sexually transmitted infections like chlamydia and gonorrhoea are a common cause of reproductive tract inflammation.

In pelvic inflammatory disease and tubal infertility, these infections trigger low-grade chronic inflammation that, over time, causes changes in uterine tissues, fallopian tubes and ovaries. These organs try to repair themselves but in doing so stiffen the tissues and cause loss of function and fertility. These issues are usually noticed for the first time during infertility investigations. Typical symptoms are abdominal pain, menstrual disturbance, changes in vaginal discharge and urine, pain during sex and fever.[26]

Fertility issues are higher in people with internal reproductive organs, but they're very common.[27] Chronic inflammation can develop at different points in people's reproductive organs. Infertility is often attributed to inflammation along the extra-testicular ducts and accessory sex organs, for example, although we don't really understand yet how this inflammation causes infertility. Even second-hand exposure to smoke kills cells that produce sperm and can lead to abnormal testicular development, DNA damage and lower sperm counts. It also causes oxidative stress-induced damage to ovaries and eggs that also drives infertility. Infertility issues affect one in four couples – between 50–120 million people – globally.[28] Treatments cost around $30,000–$40,000 for every live birth.[29]

Chronic kidney disease

Chronic inflammation in kidney disease is closely linked to poor nutrition.[30] Other factors include bacterial infections in our bloodstream from dialysis, dental issues, foot ulcers, low levels of red blood cells (anaemia), chronic infection, exposure to pollutants, smoke and lack of exercise.

People with chronic kidney disease tend to have poor appetites and lower intake of protein and calories, contributing to weight and muscle loss. As well as the usual symptoms of inflammation, they can also experience anorexia, muscle wasting and weakness.

Chronic kidney disease affects 10% of the global population. About two million patients are treated every day, mostly in the US, Germany, Italy, Japan and Brazil, with even higher numbers in India and China. It costs the US about $48 billion a year, China $56 billion, and Australia $2 billion. One million people die every year from untreated chronic kidney disease.[31]

Liver disease

Inflammation is a major part of liver disease. The initial damage can happen through an infection, the use of some medications, exposure to toxins or drinking too much alcohol over a long period of time, which causes scarring (cirrhosis). The scarring causes inflammation that makes the damage worse, sometimes to the point of becoming life-threatening.[32]

Autoimmunity can also contribute to liver disease. Obesity and diabetes are risk factors in non-alcoholic fatty liver disease and liver cancer. Hepatitis is a specific infection-induced inflammatory liver disease caused by the hepatitis virus (hepatitis A–E, especially hepatitis B and C).

Symptoms of the disease include jaundice (a yellow tinge to the skin and eyes) and liver failure. Other symptoms are nausea, fatigue, diarrhoea, confusion, breathing difficulties, rectal bleeding, abdominal and leg swelling, muscle tremors and loss of consciousness.

Liver disease affects over 120 million people. It causes two million deaths worldwide each year – one million to cirrhosis, and another million to viral hepatitis, non-alcoholic fatty liver disease and liver cancer combined.[33] Hospitalised inpatients alone cost up to $20 billion a year in the US, or $20,000 per patient.[34]

Cancers

Inflammation is thought to be a main risk factor in many types of cancer.[35] Researchers recently linked inflammation (including low-level chronic or 'smouldering' inflammation, which may not have any obvious symptoms) to up to one in five cancers.[36]

Inflammation may damage DNA, which can lead to DNA mutations that cause tumours.

Inflammation's main purpose is to promote the growth of cells that repair damage: it makes DNA replicate faster, increasing the chance of mutations and the uncontrolled growth of cells that lead to tumours and cancer.

Cancer often develops as a consequence of an inflammatory disease. People with COPD, for example, are six times more likely to develop lung cancer; colitis is strongly associated with colon cancer, and hepatitis with liver cancer. Chronic infection with Helicobacter pylori bacteria (and the chronic inflammation associated with it) is now known to cause stomach cancer, while chronic human papillomavirus infection (and the inflammation associated with it) can lead to cervical cancer. Exposure to asbestos drives mesothelioma, a lung disease, and exposure to silica is behind another lung disease, silicosis, both through the inflammatory responses they provoke.

Twenty per cent of all cancers are linked to chronic infections. Thirty per cent are linked to smoking or smoke exposure and air pollution, and 35% to diet and obesity.[37]

Cancer symptoms are different depending on where in your body the cancer is, but generally include:[38]

- fever
- fatigue
- persistent cough
- eating difficulties
- neurological issues

- skin changes and jaundice
- weight loss or gain for no obvious reason
- unexplained bleeding or bruising
- blood in the urine or stool, pain or difficulty urinating or defecating
- swelling/lumps, especially in the breasts, underarms, groin, neck and stomach.

Cancer is the second most common cause of death globally, accounting for around 10 million deaths every year. Smoking or smoke exposure, infections and poor diet are common causes.[39]

Lung cancer is the most common type of cancer, killing about 1.8 million people each year, followed by colorectal cancer (900,000 people), stomach cancer (800,000 people), liver cancer (800,000 people) and breast cancer (600,000 people).[40] In 2010, cancer treatments and care cost about $1.2 trillion worldwide.[41]

The common link between all these diseases? Inflammation!

As you can see, inflammation is an aspect of the major diseases that are all too prevalent in industrialised nations. Lifestyle is often a contributing element, with factors like smoking or smoke exposure, air pollution and poor diet making people more vulnerable to these diseases.

It's important to remember that most of these diseases don't just affect a single organ: they involve whole-body (systemic) inflammation.

They may be driven by low-level smouldering chronic inflammation that you might not even be aware of, without obvious physical symptoms.

But all hope is not lost – there are concrete changes we can all make to our diet and lifestyles that suppress these harmful inflammatory responses.

As we'll see in the next few chapters, supporting the health of our gut microbiome by enjoying a healthy diet and lifestyle is one simple but powerful way we can really help drive down unnecessary and harmful inflammation in our bodies. We can fight the signs of ageing and live longer, healthier lives with an enhanced sense of wellbeing while avoiding and treating acute and chronic disease.

At the Centenary Institute, we firmly believe prevention is better than cure. We hope this book will help persuade you that you can enjoy better physical and mental health simply by looking after your gut.

We're committed to fully understanding the basic molecular and cellular processes that drive disease. We want to find what exactly causes disease development and progression, then create and test completely new ways of preventing and treating disease based on well-understood molecular mechanisms. That way, we'll be better able to explain the new treatments we develop, to help people understand why the specific medications and treatments we advise will work for them.

A good example is probiotics. We've been told to up our intake of 'good bacteria' for a long time based on the assumed benefits of good bacteria – but we didn't really understand *how* they work.

Now we can thoroughly profile the types of bacteria in the gut and the metabolites they produce that are linked to disease features – once we know these species and their molecular changes, we can specifically target them.

In inflammatory diseases, for example, we're often low on beneficial bacteria called *Bifiidobacterium* that we know ferments fibre to produce short-chain fatty acids (SCFAs) that are anti-inflammatory. So, if we see we're low on *Bifidobacterium,* we can take probiotics and fibre to help kickstart the process that suppresses inflammation.

It seems that rather than the medicine cabinet, the path to vitality and wellbeing may well just lie on our plates!

2

How does chronic inflammation cause disease?

As we saw in chapter 1, inflammation is usually a good response, but when it becomes excessive or abnormal, it underpins a whole range of chronic diseases currently plaguing the modern world.

But inflammation isn't all bad! Inflammation is simply part of our body's natural immune response: it keeps us safe from a whole range of infections that could lead to death and helps heal us when we're hurt or injured. It's only when inflammation runs rampant and turns against us that things become nasty.

Inflammation is a natural immune system defence

Historically, the average life expectancy was less than 40 years old – a much shorter lifespan than the average today. Most people, including 25% of newborns, died from infectious diseases:

for example, lung infections like pneumonia and influenza, or gut infections like diarrheal disease.

Microbes are all around us, on us, in the air we breathe, and on everything we touch. Infections that lead to disease – known as pathogenic infections – are caused by a wide range of bacteria, viruses, fungi and parasites. Each one of those causes infection in its own specific way. Humans aren't the only ones affected by them either. All living things are.

To protect ourselves, we had to develop a system to fight off infection. It's survival of the fittest through evolution: that's where our immune systems come in. Even bacteria, insects and primitive organisms like flies, sea sponges and lampreys have immune systems.

Our immune system is a complex network of cells, tissues and organs all working together to fend off hostile intruders. In fact, humans and other higher organisms have a multi-layered immune system with two main tiers of immunity: our 'innate' immune system, and 'adaptive' or 'acquired' immunity.

Innate immunity and 'good' inflammation[42]

Most microbes are beneficial, and our bodies know what to do with them. When organisms – from primitive species right through to humans – are infected with a pathogenic (or disease-causing) microbe, our innate immune system is our first line of defence. It launches a broad range of inflammatory responses that aren't specific to that microbe. As we'll see below, this defence mechanism is critical to fighting off infection at early stages.

Our innate immune system – the one we're essentially born with – is made up of physical barriers. Our skin is a barrier, and so are the mucous membranes that line our respiratory, digestive and reproductive internal tracts.

Those mucous membranes contain cells that produce a sticky mucus, which traps microbes before they can reach our cells. When they detect a foreign particle or invader, structural cells in these membranes and our innate immune cells jump into action and set off inflammatory responses.

To initiate inflammation, structural and innate immune cells release proteins (enzymes) that destroy bacterial components. These cells are white blood cells called phagocytes ('cell eaters'). Phagocytes include neutrophils, monocytes, macrophages, eosinophils, mast cells and natural killer cells. Our white blood cells are like security guards that roam around our circulatory system: when they encounter a microbe or foreign particle, they form protrusions that envelope it, drawing it into the cell for destruction by enzymes and oxidant responses. They also set off an alarm by releasing inflammatory factors in the form of chemical signals – which in turn attract an army of other immune cells as reinforcements to destroy invading microbes.

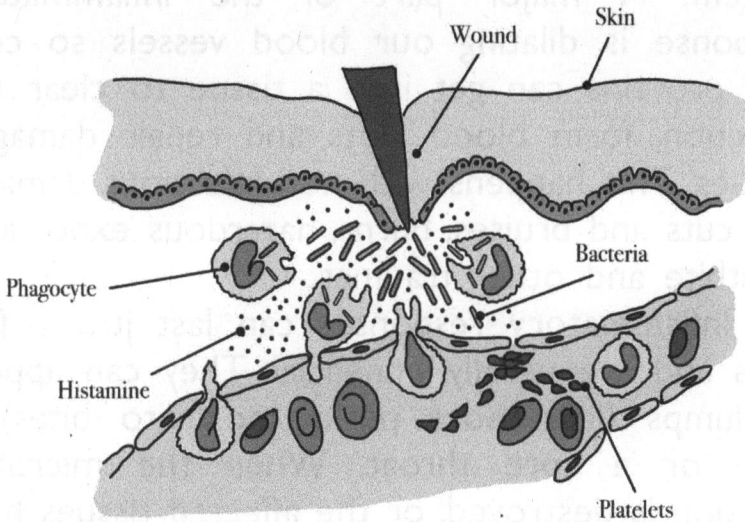

The 5 signs and symptoms of acute inflammation

Redness due to blood vessels dilating.

Heat in peripheral areas from increased blood flow and the chemical signals from inflammatory immune cells.

Swelling from fluid build-up of dilated blood vessels.

Pain from fluid build-up affecting tissue structure, and from the actions of chemical signals.

Loss of function because of swelling or pain that restricts movement.

Inflammation-related proteins and antimicrobial proteins are another part of this system. A major part of the inflammatory response is dilating our blood vessels so cells and proteins can get into a tissue to clear the infection, form blood clots and repair damaged tissues. This happens with non-infectious damage, like cuts and bruises, burns, hazardous exposures, frostbite and other traumas.

Inflammatory responses can last just a few days and are usually beneficial. They can appear as lumps (like those pesky mosquito bites), a rash or a sore throat. When the microbial invasion is destroyed, or the affected tissues have been repaired, the symptoms go away. Acute inflammation is short, sharp and purposeful: a part of our body's healing process.

Our innate immune and inflammatory responses also bring about adaptive immunity. These are all major benefits of good inflammation.

Adaptive immunity: what doesn't kill us makes us stronger

Normally, when we're exposed to infections, our innate immune system mounts a controlled inflammatory response as a first line of defence, hopefully clearing up the problem. This often brings on an 'adaptive' immune response.

During and after our bodies have fought off an infecting microbe, our immune cell responses change, creating an 'immune memory' to help us fight off the next (similar) infection more quickly and effectively. The adaptive response generates more specific responses from specific types of immune cells, T cells and B cells (lymphocytes).

B cells produce antibodies against microbial molecules they've encountered before. That's actually what getting vaccinated is all about: when we're vaccinated against a specific pathogen, 8–10 days or so later we're protected from the infection without having had it in the first place.

Once they've developed, low levels of these adaptive immune cells become permanently part of our circulating immune cells, poised to respond to any attack. When we're exposed to the same microbe again, these specific cells quickly multiply and launch a rapid (four-day) adaptive immune response that speedily and effectively clears the infection.

Infections that *aren't* cleared effectively, however, can lead to chronic inflammation, damage and potentially fatal disease.

Chronic inflammation: when things go bad

Inflammation is a two-part response: low or acute levels of threats to the immune system activate low levels of beneficial inflammation, whereas high or chronic threats activate high or prolonged levels of inflammation, which has damaging longer-term effects.

Chronic inflammation, meaning inflammation that lasts more than a few days (months or even years), happens when the initial infection or other stimulus can't be cleared effectively and the healing process is interrupted. Some infections and other foreign materials (asbestos, silica, metal and wood splinters) can't be cleared by the body's defences.

When our immune system functions well, it keeps a happy balance between tolerating harmless particles and tackling harmful intruders. An under-functioning immune system is no good because it makes us vulnerable to infection, but a hypervigilant one brings problems of its own. Our immune systems can mistake a harmless substance for a threat and over-react to it, triggering a needless inflammatory response out of proportion to the 'threat'.

When our immune system forgets to hit the off switch and goes into overdrive indefinitely, it causes chronic inflammation. The problem is, even if it's happening at a relatively low level, this constant inflammation affects body systems on a deeper internal level and doesn't display the five visible tell-tale signs of acute inflammation (see box entitled "The 5 signs and symptoms of acute inflammation").

People with underlying inflammation are predisposed to developing inflammatory diseases. The more chronic and severe the inflammation, the more long-term and severe the resulting disease – so much so that acute and/or chronic inflammation are either major drivers or major contributors to most of the prevalent diseases troubling Western societies today. These diseases develop when inflammation 'goes bad' and causes harm. When initial immune responses don't clear the initial infection or damage, a chain reaction of inflammation goes out of control.

Major features of bad chronic inflammation are excessive numbers of inflammatory cells, along with chemical signals, enzymes and oxidants that these and other cells release. Although they're designed to kill and clear infections, when inflammatory cell numbers get too high, they damage our own healthy cells and tissues, which in turn can lead to inflammatory disease.

While some infections and other foreign materials can't be cleared by the body's defences, factors like poor diet and unhealthy lifestyle choices *can* be changed.

Change doesn't need to be dreary or dramatic to benefit your health! Everyone can make changes to their diet or lifestyle in a way that works best for them: basically, you can make it fun. A fresh mango, some avocado, yoghurt or pistachios can make a great replacement snack when you're craving chips or sweets, for example. It's just as easy for me to go to the fridge for fruit rather than the cupboard for chips. It's about what *you* like and what works for you.

Inflammatory factors & modern life

Another way to look at the inflammation pandemic is through a more holistic lens, looking at the huge roles our modern lifestyle and diet play.

Our bodies are perfectly balanced with the natural world, after many millions of years of evolution and natural selection. Although our way of life has changed profoundly since the Industrial Revolution, our physiology has not. Environmental degradation on a global scale has exposed our bodies to all kinds of toxic assaults and irritants, and even affected our food chain.

Modern environmental causes of inflammation include:

- air pollution (e.g. vehicle emissions and smoke from bushfires)
- water pollution
- urbanisation and the destruction of our natural 'macro' biomes — the forests and waterways that make up our ecosystems
- microplastics and thousands of obscure chemicals in everything from processed food to personal care products (like sunscreen, make-up, shampoo and deodorant), detergents and household cleaning agents
- overuse of chemical pesticides and herbicides in farming, monoculture cropping and topsoil loss — draining the nutrients out

of farm produce and increasing its chemical load

• the use of antibiotics, hormones and steroids, all-grain diets, and 'fear killing' in factory-farmed animals

On a molecular level, our bodies recognise these compounds as being 'foreign' and trigger inflammatory responses to deal with them.

Our modern lifestyles are also wildly out of sync with our hunter-gatherer ancestors. The move away from a more physically active lifestyle to the desk-bound 9-to-5 workday, the stress and demands of the modern workplace, and the disruption of our circadian rhythms with artificial lighting all play a part in our health and disease.

But it's not all hopeless! While inflammatory triggers are all around us, and many are outside our individual control, the one thing we all *can* control is what we eat.

Enter: the gut.

The guts of it

Over the past few decades, one area that's grabbed the interest of researchers is the gut's role – specifically the trillions of teeming microbial residents that call it home – in all aspects of our health.

Our gut plays a vital role in our immune system. They help train our immune cells to distinguish between friend and foe. The chemical molecules and by-products the microbes in our gut generate help nourish us, calm our immune system and reduce our body's overall or underlying inflammation load. On the other hand, they can also set off harmful inflammatory responses, not just in the gut, but in the entire immune system network threaded throughout our body. As they say, what happens in the gut doesn't stay in the gut!

It's pretty clear that switching to a healthier, fibre-rich diet can be a very simple, but very effective, way of supporting our good gut bugs and reaping the benefits — as we'll see over the next few chapters.

3

Ageing and inflammation: inflammageing

Thanks to advances in healthcare, hygiene and living standards, we're living longer and getting older. But our longer life expectancy comes with a sharp rise in age-related chronic diseases, including arthritis, cancer, cardiovascular disease, COPD, dementia and Alzheimer's disease – chronic conditions in which, as we've seen, inflammation is a key driver. This surge in age-related inflammation has been so notable in the past few decades that it's given rise to a new term: 'inflammageing' (inflammation + ageing).

But is age-related inflammation inevitable? Are there ways we can reduce our body's underlying inflammatory load so we can slow down our inner 'inflammation clock', and in turn age healthily and well?

What is ageing?

The ageing process is easy to recognise in ourselves and others, but – surprisingly – has been difficult to define in scientific terms. Most living things change biologically over time in ways that increase the risk of death and disease and lowers our resilience to physical and environmental stresses. Most definitions of ageing (and there are many definitions) include some or all of these concepts.

Physical features, like wrinkles and grey hair, are one way to understand ageing. Or you could look at it statistically: the risk of dying increases exponentially with time, and very few people live beyond 110 years old.

Getting older is the most powerful risk factor for nearly all diseases, from emphysema or COPD, to arthritis, heart disease, dementia and cancer.

The hallmarks of ageing

The biological and cellular processes that cause ageing were extensively catalogued in 2013.[43] Called 'the hallmarks of ageing', the different cellular processes interact and cascade to cause damage to cells, organs and the whole body. Remarkably, these hallmarks of ageing have been found in most living things, from yeast to mice and worms!

The first signs of ageing start within our DNA, and the genes they encode. Over time, our DNA and protein production becomes impaired. Telomeres (a region of DNA at the tips of chromosomes that protect them from damage) become shorter. When telomeres become too short, cells stop dividing and become 'senescent' (biologically old). Senescent cells are sometimes called 'zombie cells' because they're only half alive – they don't replicate or do anything useful apart from producing substances that cause inflammation.[44] Ageing is also connected to lower stem cell numbers, which are needed to repair damaged tissues.

The last hallmark of ageing is the mechanisms that allow cells to communicate with each other: as we age, communication between cells becomes disturbed. The most important example of this hallmark is the increase in inflammation.[45]

It's possible to speed up or delay ageing just by changing a single component of the complex pathways that make up the hallmarks. (Obviously the aim is to *delay* ageing, along with the diseases and disabilities that usually accompany getting older.) In fact, it's been possible to substantially delay ageing in animals like mice, fruit flies, worms and yeast – but whether this can be translated into humans is as yet unknown.[46]

The hallmarks of ageing are all linked: when one hallmark is damaged, it often leads to changes in the other hallmarks, triggering a cascade of processes that cause and accelerate ageing. Each of the hallmarks – especially inflammation – can be considered both a cause *and* a consequence of ageing.

Our immune system has no off switch

Our immune system is constantly stimulated throughout our lives. It responds to the wide range of infectious agents (like viruses, bacteria, and other challenges) that we're exposed to, and to all the molecules, components and cells in our bodies that become damaged and degraded. The longer we live, the more our immune system is activated. This is sometimes called our 'immunobiography'.

Some infections particularly affect our immune system and how it ages. One of these is cytomegalovirus (CMV) – a virus so widespread it infects most of us by the time we're 40 years old. Although the initial infection is usually mild, CMV silently stays in our bodies for the rest of our lives, changing the function of T cells (immune cells).[47]

Old age is also associated with periodontitis, a chronic infection of the tissues around the teeth that leads to tooth loss and gum shrinkage – which is why older people are sometimes said to be 'long in the tooth'. This inflammation in the mouth has been linked with inflammation in the rest of the body.[48]

Enter again: the gut

Ageing changes our gut microbiome – the trillions of bacteria living in our digestive system.[49] Some of these bacteria, the products and metabolites they release, reduce inflammation in the rest of the body, other bacteria products and metabolites increase it. The older we get, the more inflammation-increasing bacteria and the less inflammation-reducing bacteria we have in our gut microbiome. In particular, there's less *Akkermansia* bacteria, which are usually thought to be good for health in old age.[50] The reason for these changes in gut bacteria are still unclear, but it's likely age-related changes in gut function, immunity and diet.

Our dietary habits change over time for any number of reasons: changes in income, health, marital status and so on. These changes often lead to a lower quality of diet. The foods we eat, especially foods high in fatty acids and low in anti-inflammatory nutrients, are linked to increased inflammation. It's now known that high-fat diets, especially the ones with highly processed polyunsaturated fatty acids, increase inflammation. On a molecular level, saturated fatty acids activate inflammatory responses inside our lung cells: a high trans-fat meal, for example, increases airway inflammation – a particular issue for asthma sufferers.

The rise of 'inflammageing'

So what's the effect of chronic infections, damaged cells, fatty foods, changes in microbes on our immune system and other challenges? With ageing, they lead to a state of permanent, low-grade, generalised inflammation without there being any obvious infections. This was first called inflammageing some 20 years ago, and its scientific foundations are now established.[51]

Inflammageing doesn't target any particular infection – and it doesn't mean our immune system has become better at fighting off infections and other challenges. Unfortunately, the increased inflammation that comes with old age is linked to poor responses to infections and damaged cells, tissues and organs. Some diseases, especially COPD, are thought to be a form of accelerated ageing.

Inflammageing and disease

Senescent cells (non-dividing 'zombie' cells), which accumulate with age, produce a range of proteins that exaggerate inflammageing.[52] Inflammageing has mostly been studied by measuring the blood levels of proteins called cytokines.

Interleukin-6 (IL-6)	The first (and most studied!) cytokines of this group. IL-6 is produced mainly by macrophages (large cells found in most tissues, especially the liver). It causes inflammatory responses by activating and stimulating other immune cells. It's also produced by zombie cells. IL-6 blood levels rise in age-related syndromes and diseases, including sarcopenia (decrease in muscle mass and function in old age), COPD, Alzheimer's disease, inflammatory arthritis and some cancers. Elevated IL-6 levels have almost always been found in older people who are frail.[53]

Tumour necrosis factor (TNF)	The next cytokine is TNF. Like IL-6, TNF is mainly produced by macrophages and can increase inflammation throughout the body. In some studies, it's been linked to ageing, frailty, COPD, Alzheimer's disease and some cancers.
C-reactive protein (CRP)	High levels of CRP are also linked to inflammageing. Unlike IL-6 and TNF, which are mostly measured for research purposes, CRP is commonly measured by doctors to help diagnose infections or autoimmune diseases.

There's an especially strong relationship between inflammageing and many chronic diseases.[54] For example, older people with higher blood levels of IL-6, TNF, CRP and other proteins are more likely to develop strokes, heart attacks or other cardiovascular diseases.[55]

A lot of other serious chronic diseases – emphysema/COPD, type 1 diabetes, Alzheimer's disease and cancers – show increased markers of inflammageing.[56]

All these findings point to a strong link between inflammation and chronic age-related diseases. By finding ways to reduce or control the underlying level of inflammation in our bodies, we might be able to delay the physical and cognitive decline associated with getting older so we can enjoy better health in our golden years.

What is the science telling us? The key to keeping inflammatory illness at bay is to maintain a gut-friendly diet and healthy lifestyle.

With that in mind, let's talk in more depth about gut health.

4

Welcome to the microbiome

You are what you eat

The terms microbiota and microbiome were virtually unknown until the last few decades. The more we learn about the rich, teeming jungle of microscopic bugs living in our gut, the more it seems the old adage 'you are what you eat' should be updated to the more scientifically accurate 'you *and your microbiome* are what you eat'.

Invisible to the naked eye, tiny microbes line every exposed crook and cranny of our skin, as well as our nose, urinary tract and the lining inside our gut (our entire gastrointestinal tract, from our mouth all the way down to our anus) – with different microbial communities favouring different regions.

Collectively, the distinct communities of microorganisms that jostle for space on our bodies are known as microbiota. But when we talk specifically about the community of microbes and the genes that they produce, we then use the term microbiome.

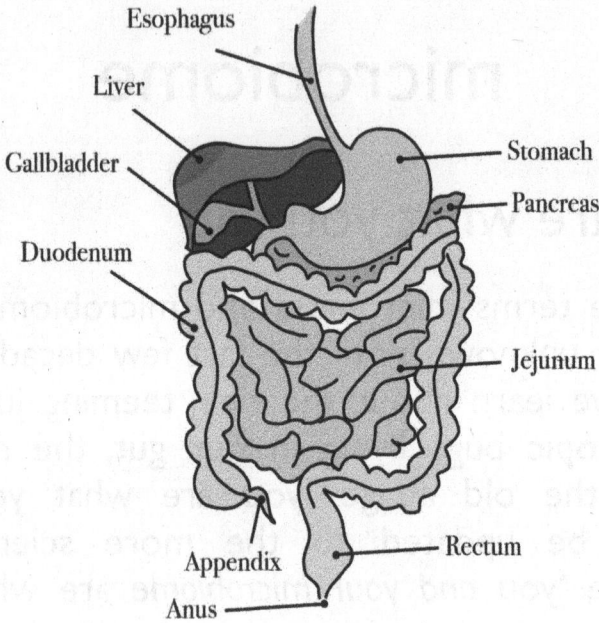

Our gut is home to more than 100 trillion microorganisms from 4000–6000 different species. We carry most of these tiny bugs in our colon – bacteria, but also yeasts, fungi, viruses, archaea and parasites.[57] Amazingly, 30% of our faeces is made up of microorganisms! Together, our gut bugs weigh as much as our brain. Some scientists even consider us hosts to a whole ecosystem of organisms, describing this symbiotic system as a 'human–microbiome superorganism'.[58]

A rich and wondrous symbiosis

Historically, microbes were seen as simply 'bad' or 'unhygienic', responsible for causing all kinds of illnesses. It's now very clear that these tiny inhabitants of our body are critical for our overall health. A lot of the microbes that share our bodies are actually beneficial – which makes sense, given we've co-evolved with our microbiome from the very beginning.[59]

All these microbes combined have far more metabolic genes than we do, meaning they can offer us unique functions our bodies can't perform by ourselves. They help us digest foodstuffs that are otherwise indigestible, for example, and make vitamins (like vitamin K and B vitamins) and other beneficial compounds our body needs. They play many roles in our metabolism, keep our immune system healthy, and even communicate information to our brains. We 'feed' them and give them a safe place to live, and they in turn nourish us. When we have enough beneficial (or at least harmless) varieties, they also provide a protective barrier against undesirable 'enemy' microbes.

This living, breathing ecosystem of microbes is in many ways controlling our physiology and our health. There are strong connections between diet and disease through the gut microbiome, and these links continue to emerge. Not surprisingly, it turns out what we eat is probably the greatest determinant of our gut microbiome's health, which is intrinsically wired into all aspects of our biology – especially our immune system.

There's evidence, for example, that taking childhood antibiotics that wipe out most of the microbiome is strongly associated with developing immune-driven allergic diseases like asthma. In fact, there's the gut–lung,[60] gut–liver, gut–brain, gut–everything axis, which describes how the gut microbiome is critical for all of our tissues to function normally.

As scientists exploring nature's intricate connections, one of the initial questions we always ask to find out if something has an important role is, 'what if we remove it?'.

A germ-free dystopia

You wake up in a germ-free world. No more bacterial infections; no more viral infections; no more fungal infections. You take a multivitamin with your breakfast and think about all the fermented and microbe-produced food you've seen in magazines of the past. Kimchi, kombucha, cheese, bread, beer, wine ... all gone since the world became germ-free.

Then you hear the news: a highly deadly virus has emerged and is spreading, killing everyone in its path. Maybe it was missed during the Great Clean? Maybe it came back on a piece of space junk? Maybe it's aliens? And now, all of humanity will fall to this virus. A virus that was once known as the common cold.

A germ-free world is more fiction than fact, but one that has captured the imagination of early scientists and the general public. Technology expanded from the initial germ-free incubators for research to plastic incubators for babies with compromised immune systems, to the 'bubble' that famously housed the Boy in the Bubble, David Vetter.[61] The ethical questions posed by such technological advances would fill books by themselves, but what's become very clear is that a host and its microbiome are deeply interconnected.

Take germ-free mice, for example. These mice are born through caesarean section into a germ-free world and are raised in microbe-free isolators.[62] In this environment, scientists can administer single or multiple strains of microbes (and/or the byproducts they produce – their 'metabolites') to investigate how they interact with their host.

Our gut and our skin are the two largest surfaces exposed to microbes. We're exposed to them in the uterus, and we get a further massive influx of microbes during and immediately after childbirth.[63] This establishes our microbiome as soon as we're born. The skin is a very harsh environment: it is nutrient poor, very dry and has a protective layer of dead cells and sweat glands that secrete urea and sweat to kill bacteria. As a result, there are only low levels of microbes on the skin. The gut on the other hand is a veritable bacterial heaven.

In germ-free animals, not being exposed to microbes has major effects. The animals don't develop normally and have many health problems. It alters the structure of their gut and their nutritional needs,[64] and affects their brain and immune cells development,[65] among other dysfunctions.[66] Germ-free animals don't have any bacteria to digest dietary fibre. There's also no bacteria to 'educate' the immune cells in the gut, which then develop to be hyperactive and hyper-responsive to any invading microbes – including harmless ones – leaving the animals vulnerable to a whole range of infectious and inflammatory diseases.[67]

It's clear from these germ-free studies that we need all the micro-flora we've co-evolved with for the healthy functioning of our bodies.

Challenges in studying the microbiome

The discovery that our gut microbiome has significant impacts on us has been one of the greatest revolutions in 21st century biomedical science. We've known for over 300 years that microorganisms live in the human gut, but their impact on our health only started to be worked out in the last decade or two, mainly thanks to technological advances. Each of us has a unique combination of trillions of bacteria in our gut, with the highest density in our colon. Our colon is home to so many bacteria it's considered one of the most complex ecosystems on Earth.

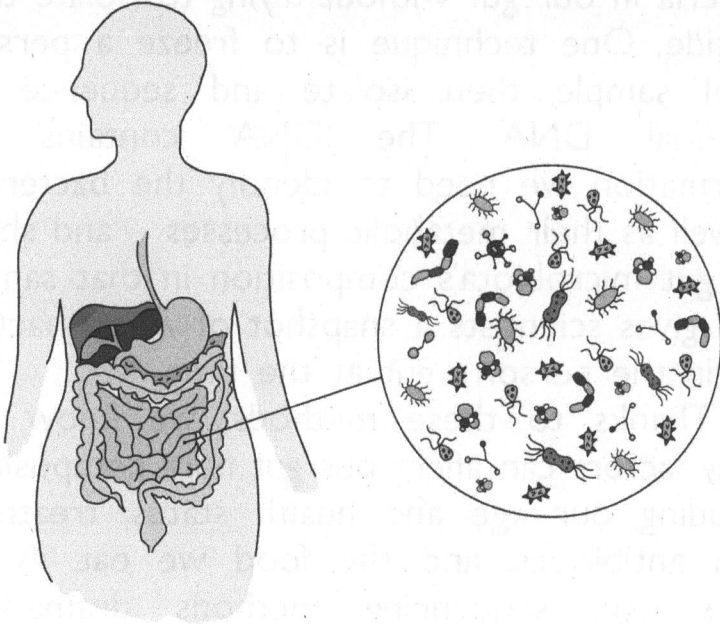

Despite their extraordinarily high numbers, it's still very challenging to study these bacteria. The first limitation is that gut bacteria normally live in an oxygen-deficient environment. They're highly sensitive to oxygen and will die when exposed to it in a laboratory. We also still don't have a clear idea of how to keep microbes alive outside the gut, in particular which nutrients they each need. Many bacteria are still poorly known – or even yet to be discovered – and they all have different needs and properties. It's impossible to culture all these thousands of bacteria at once.

Instead, different techniques have been developed to study the presence or absence of bacteria in our gut without trying to isolate them outside. One technique is to freeze a person's stool sample then isolate and sequence the bacterial DNA. The DNA contains the information we need to identify the bacteria – as well as their metabolic processes – and shows the gut microbiota's composition in that sample. This gives scientists a snapshot of which bacteria are in the person's gut at the time.

Thanks to these methods, we know that many factors can affect our gut flora composition, including our age and health status, treatment with antibiotics, and the food we eat. A few years ago, sequencing methods dramatically improved, and we now know which bacteria are present in our bodies and what they do. We can work out whether they can produce specific products, if they can metabolise therapeutic drugs, and if they can digest particular types of food.

What do our gut bugs tell us?

Our gut microbiota is now a thoroughly researched field in science – but why do we care so much?

As we've seen, studies on germ-free mice have given us major insights into how gut bacteria can affect their bodies. Kept under strictly sterile conditions, these mice have numerous immune, metabolic and behavioural defects, showing that the gut microbiota influences their organ development and function.[68]

These germ-free mice have also helped us understand how specific types of bacteria can interact with the body. When certain bacteria are administered to their gut, a particular immune cell missing in the germ-free mice is restored. This means specific gut bacteria can send signals to the body and affect the function of immune cells.[69]

It's been suggested that your microbiome does a better job of predicting obesity than your genes. If the gut microbiota from obese mice is isolated and administered to germ-free mice, the germ-free mice become overweight and develop metabolic diseases.[70] In an intriguing North American study, researchers transplanted stool microbes from human female twins to germfree mice. Even though the mice ate the same diet, the mouse that got the obese twin's stool microbes became obese, while the mouse that got the lean twin's microbes stayed lean.[71] The obese mouse also developed several associated metabolic alterations.

A big critique in biomedical research is that mice aren't humans – which is true, but there are a lot of similarities between human and animal gut microbiota. The main family of gut bacteria in humans, *Bacteroidetes* and *Firmicutes*, are the same in mice. This is why gut bacteria from humans can be used to recolonise a mouse gut.

One human study involving 800 people found that their individual gut microbiome influences each person's unique blood sugar response after eating the exact same foods.[72] With this information, researchers used each volunteer's gut microbe profile to predict which foods would cause less of a blood sugar spike. They found each person had a completely individual response to the food, which they concluded was a reflection of their microbial profile.

Changes in the gut microbiota have been seen in most diseases including allergies, autoimmune diseases, cancer, COPD and metabolic diseases,[73] but at this stage we still don't know whether these changes are a *cause* or a *consequence* of the disease – probably both.

Our gut bacteria and our body, especially our immune system, interact with and influence each other. Under healthy conditions, there's a balance in which the gut microbiota have a healthy composition and the immune system behaves normally. But when one part of the balance is disrupted, the other part is as well.

Our immune system becomes over-activated when we have a disease, and releases products that can affect our gut microbiota community. Antibiotic treatment also disrupts our gut microbiota, which means our immune system doesn't function as it should. This can lead to disease development.[74] As we've mentioned, studies show that over-using antibiotics in young children is strongly linked to the development of allergies and asthma.

Microbe 'ecosystems': fluid yet stable

In simple terms, a microbiome is a community of microorganisms (bacteria, fungi, viruses) that maintains its 'structure' in a defined ecological boundary or habitat. Ecological communities are dynamic; since their boundaries are leaky, organisms and resources can move in or out of the ecosystem.[75]

In healthy people, although the gut microbiome changes from day to day, the community 'structure' resists major change.[76] If a gut disturbance is more than the community's ability to resist change, fluctuations in the microbiome structure will happen – but when the disturbance is removed, the microbiome tends to bounce back to how it was, showing a certain resilience.[77]

If we track people's microbiomes over time, we can see consistent differences between different individuals,[78] which can help us understand how our microbiome influences our risk of disease.

Our microbiome is dynamic, and individually distinct

So we know the idea that microbes are either 'good' or 'bad' is an oversimplification. Instead, how our microbes behave depends on their environment (much like us humans!). For example, when *Clostridium difficile* (*C. diff*) causes problems, it can lead to symptoms ranging from mild to life-threatening. And yet, *C. diff* is part of the normal microbiota in our intestines: our microbiome's more dominant members often suppress its growth.[79] Similarly, other bacterial members, like *E. coli* and *Bacteroides*,[80] can cause severe illness if they travel outside the gut into our bloodstream or tissues, but when they're in the colon, these bacteria can offer important contributions to our health.

In many cases, our microbes are better at digesting and unpacking our foods than we are. Our food is also *their* food, and like us, each of them has its own distinctive food preferences. So if you don't give them the nutrients they need (e.g. by removing an entire food group, or not eating enough of certain foods) you could starve elements of your microbiota, making crucial species go extinct.

Although our microbes do work together, each provides its own unique effects. While there can be some similarities, if certain microbes are lost, so too is the community's potential to have a particular effect.

Clostridioides difficile (C. diff)

A bacteria that causes diarrhea and inflammation in the colon, and may also cause colon cancer.

Generally speaking, greater microbial diversity is linked to beneficial effects. The more diverse your gut microbiota is, the more skills your individual microbe community is likely to have.

And here's the really exciting thing: unlike our own human genes, our microbiome can be changed. When people are born with a genetic defect, that defect is there for the rest of their lives, but we are not stuck with our microbiome. If you change what you do or eat today, your microbiota will be different tomorrow. This means we have the potential to alter our microbiome – for better or worse.

5

How our gut microbiome influences inflammation

The gut's main purpose is to absorb nutrients and distribute them around the body, where they can be put to use. It makes sense, then, that anything the bacteria in our gut produces will inevitably be transported around our bodies as well.

Our gut microbes eat whatever we do: the microbes break foodstuffs down into smaller products called metabolites. With their general and specific nutrient requirements, bacteria produce their own set of by-products (or metabolites) during their own biological processes. These microbial metabolites are small enough to be used by our intestinal cells or absorbed into our blood circulation. Metabolites have a broad impact on our body, beyond just our gut.

Our immune system responds to microbial metabolites

Not all bacterial products interact with our body in the same way. Our cells can sense the metabolites produced by bacteria, because they have specific receptors that are activated by them. Different bacteria produce different by-products – some of which can cause inflammation while others reduce it.

Microbiota

The collective term for the different distinct microorganism communities in our gut (including bacteria, viruses, fungi and other organisms).

The immune system needs to monitor the presence of microbes and make a decision as to tolerating them if they are in the right place (and doing the right thing) and reacting aggressively if they cross those boundaries. It does this primarily using distinctive structural components of microbial cells that are not found in animal cells – we call these MAMPs. They provide easily recognisable signals that induce inflammation by activating receptors on the cells lining our gut, or the immune cells in our blood and tissues (e.g. macrophages), which normally protect our tissues against infection.

When they're activated, these receptors send a signal to our immune system that a bad bacteria (pathogen) is in the wrong place, ringing alarm bells and stimulating an inflammatory response. Blood vessels dilate, chemical inflammatory signals (cytokines and chemokines) are produced, inflammatory and immune cells flood the area, and anti-microbial factors like defensins and oxidants are released.

This is arguably the most important part of the interactions between our gut microbiome and inflammation. When our immune system detects factors produced by our gut bugs and sees them as 'foreign', it triggers an inflammatory response to help eliminate them.

This is how changes in the composition of our gut microbiota can either contribute to inflammatory processes or calm down excessive inflammation.

Short-chain fatty acids (SCFA) are the most characterised byproduct released by our gut bacteria. They affect our immune system and induce the production of regulatory T-cells, which are anti-inflammatory and play an important role in controlling inflammation.

Lower numbers of regulatory T-cells are often found in people with allergies, asthma,[81] and autoimmune diseases like multiple sclerosis, rheumatoid arthritis and type I diabetes. Interestingly, experimental studies show that increasing our production of short-chain fatty acids has a beneficial effect on these diseases.

As we saw in chapter 2, inflammation can be a healthy, protective and lifesaving response to infection. But when our inflammation and immune responses are over-activated, it can lead to inflammatory diseases in the gut (as well as affect many organs and tissues beyond the gut), contributing to a lot of the chronic inflammatory health conditions we introduced in chapter 1.

Maintaining immune tolerance with symbiotic bugs

When we're healthy, our immune system is tolerant and doesn't react to the normal, benign things we're regularly exposed to. It only reacts to dangerous intruders, like pathogens.

Tolerant immunity is maintained through the combined efforts of our internal gut mucus barrier and a healthy microbiome. The mucus layer – especially in our large intestine, where most bacteria live – can be an effective barrier to stop immune responses getting over-activated. Bacterial species that usually dominate a healthy microbiome are known as symbiotic bacteria: that is, bacteria which normally live in the microbiome without hurting us or causing disease.

An important feature of these bacteria, like the *Prevotella* species, is that their components are less able to activate our inflammatory responses, so they can survive closer to the surface of our guts. They take up the available space and protect against more dangerous bacteria.

These and other symbiotic bacteria (e.g. *Faecalibacterium*, *Bifidobacterium*, *Lactobacillus*, *Clostridium*, *Bacteroides*) also produce anti-inflammatory products and metabolites that help calm down our immune system and maintain a tolerant environment.

These products include short-chain fatty acids (produced when bacteria ferments dietary fibre in our gut)[82] and indole compounds (produced when bacteria metabolise the amino acid tryptopha).[83] These anti-inflammatory compounds induce immune tolerance that allows the bacteria to live close to our gut's surface without causing an inflammatory response to get rid of them.

Our good gut bugs feast on fibre

Researchers have studied dietary fibre's beneficial effects on our gut health and general wellbeing. We know developed nations eat high levels of processed foods, sugar and fat, and only half the recommended daily intake of dietary fibre – a diet that's been linked to a dramatic increase in cardiovascular diseases, as well as allergic and inflammatory conditions like inflammatory bowel disease, asthma and diabetes.

So, researchers looked at whether adding fibre back into the diet might help prevent disease, or at least make diseases less severe. Short answer: it works! Including more fibre in your diet is linked to lower blood pressure,[84] and a reduced risk of asthma, rectal cancer,[85] cardiovascular diseases,[86] diabetes[87] and breast cancer.[88]

Of course, humans can't actually digest dietary fibre – but a bunch of helpful microbes can. This is where the microbiome comes in.

We now know that some bacteria (like *Lactobacillus*, *Prevotella* and *Bifidobacterium* species) feed on dietary fibre.[89] A high fibre intake is associated with an increase of these fibre-loving microbes,[90] which also have anti-inflammatory effects in our body.[91] So when we're consuming dietary fibre, we're really feeding the bacteria in our gut that help keep our gut and the rest of our bodies healthy and well.

Dr Clare Bailey's Nutrition Tip #1

Most of us eat less than half the recommended amount and variety of fibre. Aim to eat 25–30 grams of fibre a day to support a healthy gut microbiome, including the three main types of fibre:

• **Insoluble fibre** is coarse and scratchy. It's found in most vegetables, fruits, beans, pulses, nuts and seeds, providing bulk to keep things moving in your digestive tract.

• **Soluble fibre** is more of a gel texture, which is highly fermentable and supports beneficial bacteria. It's particularly found in oats, barley and psyllium husks, as well as vegetables like parsnips, okra, eggplant, peas, beans and onions. Some fruits like pears, mango, apples and oranges also provide soluble fibre, as do nuts and seeds.

- **Resistant starch,** which usually gets completely fermented, encourages the beneficial microbes that in turn produce substances to protect and support gut health (instead of simply being released as sugars). Resistant starch is usually found in foods such as whole grain cereals, especially in oats and barley. Other sources include beans and legumes, including peas, black beans and soybeans. Some resistant starch is also produced in the cooking process, when starchy foods like pasta, potatoes or bread is cooked and allowed to cool before eating, reducing the amount of starch absorbed when eaten.

Getting enough fibre is important for heart and metabolic health, along with reducing inflammation, improving immunity and even improving mood. Take it slowly when increasing fibre, though, as you may suffer from wind!

Short-chain fatty acids: soothing the inflammatory beast

Dietary fibre is broken down into three main short-chain fatty acids: butyrate, acetate and propionate.

Butyrate

Butyrate is produced by bacteria like *Faecalibacterium prausnitzii*, which can live close to our gut surface. It has many beneficial effects. It's easily absorbed by our gut cells and is a major source of energy. It also strengthens connections between the individual cells in our gut wall, keeping it strong against foreign particles: when our gut wall is damaged (known as 'leaky gut'), bacteria and other harmful particles can get into tissues and trigger inflammation.[92] Butyrate is anti-inflammatory and suppresses inflammation.

Acetate

The most produced short-chain fatty acid is acetate; it also circulates in our bloodstream.[93] Acetate stops an inflammatory response from being activated by being bound by receptors (GPCRs) to control inflammation, which can be important to controlling gut and other inflammation levels.

Propionate

One study has shown that giving propionate to patients with multiple sclerosis can reduce the severity of their disease.[94] Feeding our gut microbiome a diet that helps the symbiotic bacteria in our gut flourish means they can keep producing these beneficial short-chain fatty acids, which helps prevent and treat disease, modulate our immune responses and maintain our health.

A lot of research has looked at *how* short-chain fatty acids prevent inflammation. One way they work is through the receptors on immune cell surfaces (G-coupled protein receptors, or GPRs).

Short-chain fatty acids bind to the immune cells using a range of these receptors (GPR41, GPR43 and GPR109), telling them to produce fewer inflammatory and more anti-inflammatory signals, which helps calm inflammatory responses in those and other nearby cells as well. If we remove these GPR receptors in animals, their immune cells become hyperactive and stop working properly, making inflammation and inflammatory diseases worse. Scientists can now develop drugs that stimulate these receptors to induce anti-inflammatory effects.[95]

Gut dysbiosis: the root of many problems?

The fact that some bacteria are beneficial shows how deeply connected our gut microbiome is to our health. We know the link between low fibre intake and many allergic and inflammatory diseases is an out-of-balance gut microbiome – a micro-flora imbalance known as dysbiosis.

Dysbiosis

Dysbiosis happens when our gut ecosystem is out of balance. It is involved in a range of digestive disturbances and is closely linked to many inflammatory diseases. Being ill or chronically stressed can contribute to dysbiosis, but poor diet is a major cause. Improving our diet and lifestyle can help bring our gut flora community and their interactions with our own cells and tissues back into balance.

Just as some microbes break down our food into helpful *anti-inflammatory* compounds like short-chain fatty acids, other microbes produce *pro-inflammatory* by-products. Dysbiosis occurs with different allergic and inflammatory conditions, including inflammatory bowel disease,[96] as well as asthma, cardiovascular diseases,[97] chronic obstructive pulmonary disease[98] and mental illnesses.[99] Changes to the metabolites produced by our gut flora are also increasingly linked to various inflammatory conditions.[100]

Immune tolerance

When your immune system is tolerant, it doesn't react to your body's own antigens. It's actively unresponsive to cells that could potentially start an immune response.

More specifically, the metabolites produced by our gut bacteria can regulate our immune tolerance. Dysbiosis in the gut and elsewhere can cause inflammation, which can lead to chronic inflammatory disease.

The onset of disease, use of antibiotics (which can also deplete the number of good bugs in our microbiome) or a breakdown of the mucus barrier that normally protects the lining of our gut can all cause disturbances to the microbiome.

In a healthy gut, competition between bacteria species for nutrients and space allows symbiotic bacteria to live closest to our gut lining. But when you have a disease, a small number of symbionts that are not working properly or more damaging bacteria gain a selective advantage and outcompete other more beneficial bacteria and disrupt good interactions with our cells and tissues. You end up with fewer bacteria species, but more or less bacteria overall – usually due to the increased growth of a small number of species that dominate the microbiome.[101] This over-stimulates the body's immune responses, giving rise to inflammation.

Tolerant immune responses are also essential in preventing food allergies and asthma. In the case of food allergies, immune tolerance helps stop excessive inflammation in response to normally non-threatening foodstuffs like eggs, nuts or gluten. Excessive immune responses to things like pollen, house dust mites or dust can trigger asthma and hay fever.

Even a small change in our microbiome can have a snowball effect. Inflammation and damage to the gut creates an opportunity for more 'bad' bacteria to grow. This ultimately leads to an imbalance in the microbiome and its interaction with us (dysbiosis) as these bad bacteria species take more and more space, resulting in a loss of immune tolerance and chronic inflammation.

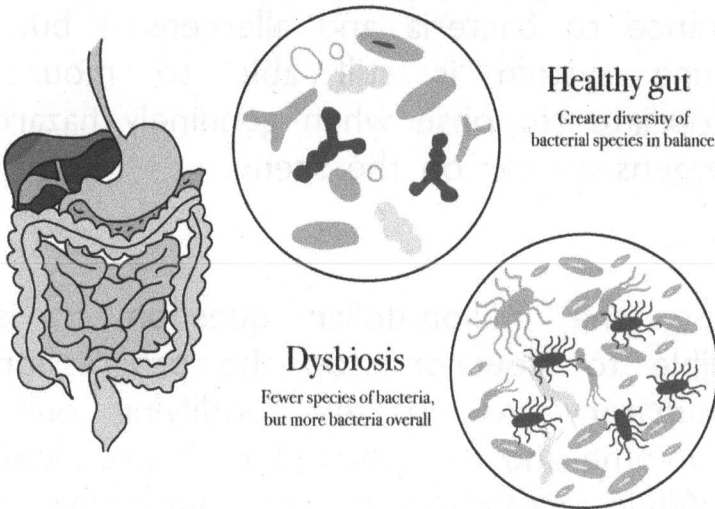

Healthy gut
Greater diversity of bacterial species in balance

Dysbiosis
Fewer species of bacteria, but more bacteria overall

Food for thought

The food we eat can change our microbiome's composition and the metabolism of the different bacterial species in our microbiome. Diet is a major factor in controlling which bacterial products our bodies are exposed to, which can have big consequences for our inflammatory state.

Symbiotic relationship

A relationship in which organisms (bacteria, people, other things) exist together in a way that benefits everyone.

A healthy microbiome exists in a symbiotic relationship with our immune system. This co-existence gives our bodies a certain level of tolerance to bacteria and allergens – but our immune system is still able to mount an appropriate response when genuinely hazardous pathogens appear on the scene.

So, the million-dollar question is, is it possible to slow or stop the progression of inflammatory diseases by modifying our gut microbiome and the metabolites it produces?

While researchers are busy untangling all the important microbes, metabolites and microbiome modifications that may help counter the modern epidemic in inflammatory conditions, we at the Centenary Institute believe prevention is better than cure.

These days, it's well accepted that a diverse, fibre-rich diet with less processed foods nourishes and promotes the growth of a diverse microbiome. Diversity is important: it'd be unwise to completely eliminate particular nutrient groups from a normal diet. A healthy lifestyle that includes a well-balanced diet is a sensible way to help promote and maintain your microbiome's health – and changing your diet doesn't have to be hard!

6

How diet shapes our microbiome

We're still discovering just how deeply integrated our microbiome is with all our bodily systems. We know that when we don't take care of our gut microbiome, we start to notice signs of dysfunction in our tissues, organs and body overall, and experience symptoms of allergic and inflammatory diseases.

Global modernisation brought an epidemic of lifestyle-related chronic diseases like cardiovascular disease, diabetes, asthma and allergies. The causes and symptoms of each disease are different, but the one recurring link between all of them is diet.

Our microbiome is hungry!

A good diet is crucial for good health. It's estimated that more than one in five deaths worldwide can be attributed to poor diet.[102]

A lot of the health consequences of a poor diet are linked to the microbiome. Remember, our bodies are home not just to human cells, but microbes (with at least comparable cell numbers) as well.[103]

Our gut wall and mucous membranes are a physical barrier that separates 'us' from the microbiome that lives on and inside us. As we saw in the last chapter, our gut microbiome feeds on the same food we eat, breaking the foodstuffs down into metabolites (like beneficial short-chain fatty acids) that are important for our health.

Bacterial communities need a supply of nutrients to function and reproduce. Without nutrients, they won't work the way they're meant to. Carbohydrates and fats supply bacteria with the energy and components they need to build the structural parts of their cells. Amino acids are needed to make proteins, and micronutrients (like vitamins and minerals) are used in chemical reactions performed by bacterial cells.

Gut bugs are picky eaters

There are about 4000–6000 bacteria species in our gut. Incredibly, each species has its own specific nutritional needs, and produces its own particular metabolites ('breakdown' or waste products). So, the nutrients we feed ourselves can make a big difference to our gut bacteria's ability to survive and multiply.[104]

Some bacteria, like the *Proteobacteria* family, are pro-inflammatory – they produce toxins and metabolites that cause inflammation in our body. Some of these bacteria don't have the enzymes they need to digest complex carbohydrates, so instead they use (or metabolise) simple sugars for energy to survive, grow and produce their metabolites. Some bacteria can't produce their own specific vitamins or amino acids, needing them to be present in the gut instead.[105]

For some bacterial species, particular nutrients give them a disproportionate survival advantage. The antioxidant vitamins C and E, for example, help anaerobic bacteria survive. The *Bacteroides* species can't survive in environments of high oxidative stress — an imbalance between oxidants and antioxidants.

It's a jungle in there

The different bacterial species in our microbiome are in constant competition with each other. They often release components and metabolites that kill or slow the growth of their competitors. Many bacteria even produce their own antibiotics — including some of the antibiotics we use today to treat infections!

When thinking about our overall health, it's not just about making sure enough nutrients are being supplied to our microbiome, but that the right nutrients are supplied and in the right quantities.

This makes it possible to change our dietary habits to improve our gut health. We can provide nutrients that support the growth of the good bacteria — and we can restrict access to nutrients that the more pro-inflammatory bacteria depend on.

Boom or bust: how diet drives our microbe dynamics

The structure of the microbe community that develops in our gut depends on bacteria's ability to find a spot and establish a sustainable population there. The total of all microbe populations present in the gut determines the microbiome's structure. Microbial growth rate depends on which nutrients we feed them: diet is one way we can control their growth.

Changes in our bowel habits and defecation rate will also change the rate microbes are removed from our gut. For example, when you have diarrhea, the electrolyte balance and pH levels in your gut change, which changes how quickly bacteria is cleared from the gut as well. This is especially helpful when the diarrhea is a response to a gut infection. Limiting nutrients can also lower or prevent microbe growth. So our diet influences both the growth *and* death rates of our microbial friends.

It follows, then, that different nutrient ratios in our diet will drive different microbial responses in our gut.

Who's feeding who?

Bacteria in our gut also help supply nutrients to our own cells through two main metabolic pathways.

First, microbes use dietary fibre (carbohydrate molecules that we can't otherwise digest) as their major carbon and energy source. Using, or metabolising, dietary fibre produces short-chain fatty acids (e.g. acetate, propionate and butyrate), which our gut absorbs as nutrients. Some scientists think 6–10% of our calorie intake is from microbial fermentation processes (and up to 70% in herbivorous animals).[106]

Second, microbes create many different molecules as they grow. Their by-products include essential vitamins and amino acids that may otherwise be lacking or absent in our diet.[107] Microbes substantially enrich the nutritional quality of the food we eat. This close relationship between our gut microbes and what we eat has big implications for how our diet affects our physiology and overall health.

Besides nourishing us, microbes are also essential for our immune system. From the moment we are born, we're exposed to trillions of them, stimulating the development of our infant immune system development. Throughout our lives, the maturation of specialised immune cells in our body is influenced by microbial signals from the gut[108] – emphasising again that what we feed our gut bacteria also affects our immune system's health.

From feast to famine

It's easy to oversimplify the word *diet*. When we look at the relationship between diet and our microbiome, and how diet can drive changes in microbial communities, we need to keep in mind how multiple diet dimensions can influence our health over time.

We know we need food to fuel each of our bodily functions and meet all our nutrient requirements. But it's a bit more complicated than that.

Our food contains complex nutrient mixtures, and it's inevitable that we're going to consume multiple nutrients simultaneously. Not all nutrients are needed in the same amount though; different foods contain different nutrients, and certain foods aren't always available, all of which makes meeting our energy and nutrient demands pretty challenging.

We get around this by eating meals made up of multiple different foods at different times. Our bodies have evolved to make up for the variation in what food is available to us and the nutrients we feed ourselves.

Our physiology and metabolism adapted over time to deal with both food scarcity and food abundance – the classic case of *famine* and *feast* – making sure that our cells and tissues have a steady supply of nutrients, despite how regularly (or not) we eat. Our bodies have the amazing ability to create nutrients we don't get from eating, efficiently remove toxins to prevent buildup, and store any extra energy in various cells and tissues to draw on when calorie intake is lower.

In other words, our metabolism is highly responsive to diet – especially to deficiencies, but also to oversupply – as we'll see a little later in this chapter.

Diet, dysbiosis and chronic disease

Because we've evolved to deal with fluctuations in our food supply – and by extension, to variations in both the quantity and quality of our nutrient intake – we can think of *diet* as a pattern of food intake over different time frames.

Even short-term changes in diet can cause changes in our physiology.[109] In a cell or tissue, for example, hormone release and gene expression changes which affect our metabolism can happen within minutes. This is essential for fine-tuning things like our blood glucose concentration level, which needs to be kept in a narrow, stable range to keep our cells functioning properly. At the other extreme, long-term diet patterns are also a major risk factor for developing a range of chronic diseases.[110] Changes to our body make-up and functioning (e.g. building up fat stores) or changes in our epigenetic state (see chapter 7) can take weeks, months or even years.

Many chronic diseases can be thought of as maladaptive states, meaning underlying processes (like chronic inflammation) are keeping our bodies in an unhealthy state.[111] As we've seen, it's now believed that changes to our microbiome are involved in this unhealthy state and contribute to disease.

We can see this maladaptive state in chronic intestinal inflammation. People with chronic intestinal inflammation have a higher level of pro-inflammatory microbes in their microbiomes compared to healthy people.[112] The microbe community adapts by favouring organisms that can tolerate living in an inflamed gut environment – and if the by-products (metabolites) they release are also pro-inflammatory, those microbes keep the gut in a vicious circle of inflammation, effectively maintaining a state of inflammation in an endless positive feedback loop.[113]

Nutrients big and small

Human diets across the world are very different, but once our food is broken down by our digestive processes, our cells and the microbes in our gut recognise similar individual chemical components. So while we often think of our diet in terms of 'meat, vegetables, bread and sweets', it can be more helpful to think about our broader nutritional needs instead.

Generally speaking, our diets are made up of macronutrients and micronutrients. Macronutrients make up the bulk of our diet – carbohydrates, dietary fibre, fats and proteins – and we need a lot of them. Micronutrients – vitamins and minerals – are only needed at very low levels.

Many common fast foods and snacks have damaging effects on us: processed sugars, excess saturated fats, excess alcohol, are examples. The Western diet's high intake of unhealthy fats has been linked to many inflammatory diseases, including asthma and metabolic and cardiovascular diseases. This higher fat consumption has also been linked to higher numbers of less desirable *Alistipes* and *Bacteroides* gut bacteria, and lower numbers of the anti-inflammatory *Faecalibacterium*.[114] A similar trend is observed in laboratory animals, with a high-fat diet increasing numbers of *Bacteroides* and *Bilophila,* and decreasing beneficial *Lactobacillus, Bifidobacterium* and *Akkermansia* species.[115]

Poor diet can drive many of these damaging changes in the microbiome. Even a short-term poor diet can have long-lasting effects on our microbiome's composition and subsequent inflammation. Our microbiomes need a healthy balance to function properly: too many or too few nutrients can have dramatic effects on our bodies.

> ## Dr Clare Bailey's Nutrition Tip #2
>
> What is real food? 'If it's a plant, eat it. If it's made in a plant, don't!' recommends Michael Pollan, professor of Science and Environmental Journalism at the University of California, Berkeley. He also advises people to 'Eat real food. Not too much. Mostly plants.' Aim to avoid industrially produced foods – you can often identify these by checking that you actually recognise the names of the ingredients and that it doesn't contain a long list of ingredients.

Micronutrients and the microbiome

Micronutrients are essential for many important processes in cells (both our own, and in bacterial cells) even though they're only needed in trace quantities. Because of this, changes in micronutrient intake can affect our microbiome's composition, the by-products our bacteria create, and how well our microbes cooperate with us.

Antioxidant vitamins, like vitamins C and E, can help symbiotic bacteria that are anaerobic – meaning they need low-oxygen conditions, which is normally the case in a healthy gut – to survive and thrive, especially during periods of intense oxidative stress like during acute or chronic inflammation.

Mitochondria are the engine-rooms of our cells: it's possible they were once actually bacteria that've been incorporated into the cells of all higher organisms over many millions of years. You might remember from high school biochemistry that all our cells use energy to produce new lipids, carbohydrates and proteins (among other things) to function and grow.

Adenosine triphosphate (ATP)

An energy-carrying molecule found in the cells of all living things. It's our cells main energy source – ATP captures chemical energy from food molecule breakdown and releases it to fuel other cellular processes.

There are two processes that produce ATP in cells: oxidative phosphorylation in mitochondria, and glycolysis in cytoplasm (the semi-fluid liquid that fills the inside of a cell).

In oxidative phosphorylation, electrons are passed down a 'transport train' from one molecule to another, and energy released in these electron transfers is used to form an electrochemical gradient. The energy stored in the gradient is used to make ATP.

Oxygen sits at the end of the transport chain, where it accepts electrons. This is why we need to breathe – when you're not getting enough oxygen, electrons won't be able to pass to oxygen, the electron transport chain will stop running and ATP won't be produced (and if the train stops running long enough, you die). The addition of electrons to oxygen produces oxygen radicals, which our antioxidant responses control.

When things like smoke, allergens, or fatty acids stress our cells, it damages the mitochondria, causing an over-production of oxygen radicals and oxidative stress. This activates inflammation.

Glycolysis (the process in which glucose is broken down) also creates ATP. It's quicker than oxidative phosphorylation, but less efficient. Glycolysis produces pro-inflammatory factors (IL-1b) and reduces anti-inflammatory factors (IL-10). When our cells are stressed, glycolysis works better than oxidative phosphorylation but produces more inflammatory responses.

Iron is essential to many enzymes that carry out critical roles like energy production. Unlike most other micronutrients, iron doesn't dissolve in water or our bodily fluids – it needs to be attached to something. We have special proteins (transferrin and haeme) that bind iron and transport it around.

Low iron intake makes bacteria (like *Escherichia coli*) produce more molecules that capture iron (called siderophores). Our microbiome can get more iron as a result – but at the cost of lowering the amount of iron available to us when our dietary iron intake is already low. On the other hand, if our iron intake is too high, it reduces bacterial competition close to the gut wall, which leaves space for mucus-degrading bacteria species (*Bacteroides, Proteobacteria, Verrucomicrobia*) to grow and damages the mucus barrier, leading to gut and whole-body inflammation.[116]

Excessive salt intake can damage our microbiome's ability to produce anti-inflammatory short-chain fatty acids[117] and indole products. These anti-inflammatory factors drive production of specific cells (called regulatory T cells) that control many inflammatory responses.[118]

Changes in the levels of B vitamins (including folate, thiamine and riboflavin) don't really seem to affect the composition of our microbiome, thanks to a process called 'cross-feeding' where some bacteria (e.g. *Eubacterium hallii* and *Anaerostipes caccae*) can make their own B vitamins. These vitamins are then available to other members of the microbiome that can't produce their own.

Excess macronutrients and inflammation

Being overweight or obese is associated with changes in our microbiome, leaky gut and whole-body inflammation – possibly because when we overeat, we take in more macronutrients (i.e. protein, carbohydrates and fat) than we need, reducing competition between all the different gut bacteria species. With less competition, the healthy bacteria that can cooperate with us have less of an advantage, and more pro-inflammatory bacteria grow.[119]

Our microbes can meet most of their growth needs when they have sources of carbon and nitrogen.[120] They tend to get these nutrients from our food rather than make them – so microbes that are better at foraging for their dietary nutrients are the ones that'll grow.[121]

In a classic study of genetically obese mice, researchers noticed that when they increased the mice's calorie intake while keeping their intake of other nutrients the same, the amount of *Firmicutes* bacteria in their gut went up, at the expense of *Bacteroidetes* species.[122] Other studies found that adding cellulose to the diet (to bring down the food's overall energy density and reduce the calorie intake) led to an increase in microbes (e.g. *Bacteroidetes*) that are better at using resources, like nitrogenous wastes (urea) or mucus,[123] at the expense of foraging microbes like *Firmicutes*.[124] So, even the overall calorie content of our diet can affect the growth of bacteria in our individual microbiome.

Of the three macronutrients in our diet – fat, protein and carbohydrates – fat has the least effect on microbes, since it's a very minor source of carbon and energy in an oxygen-deprived environment like the gut.[125]

But a high-fat diet *can* affect microbial diversity, mostly by diluting the proportion of protein and carbohydrate, our microbes' main energy sources.[126] A high-fat diet is effectively calorie restriction – but not for us, for our microbes! While high-fat diets reduce diversity and increase bacterial load in the gut, as well as creating the leaky gut syndrome linked to whole-body inflammation,[127] it's actually our protein and carbohydrate intake that have the biggest effects.

Comparing animal-based foods to plant-based foods, the quality of both their protein and fat are different. Animal protein, for example, doesn't have plant polysaccharides (including fibre) and has higher saturated fat levels. Eating a diet high in animal protein increases our levels of mucus-degrading bacteria.[128] These effects, along with bile profile changes, may also contribute to the microbiome differences we see between diets rich in either unsaturated or saturated fats.[129]

Dietary protein is made up of amino acids, which contain nitrogen (a key component for our symbiotic bacteria). Bacteria, like the *Akkermansia* species which are mainly anti-inflammatory and cooperate with us to limit inflammation, have more room to grow when protein intake is low. There's less of these bacteria in people with severe asthma, for example, and giving *Akkermansia* to mice reduces lung inflammation and wheezing.[130]

Studies on protein-rich diets have shown that animal-based protein increases inflammatory bacterial species (e.g. *Alistipes*, *Bacteroides* and *Bilophila*), while plant-based proteins increase beneficial bacterial species and produce more health-promoting short-chain fatty acids.[131]

Red meat and processed meat have also been linked to a higher risk of cardiovascular disease.[132] In animal studies, a high-protein diet increased potentially harmful *Escherichia*, *Enterococcus* and *Streptococcus* strains, and reduced bacteria that's good for health, like *Akkermansia*, *Ruminococcus* and *Faecalibacterium*.[133]

The difficulty with dietary detail

In nutritional research, it's difficult to isolate the effect of specific dietary components. People who eat a plant protein-rich diet might enjoy better health because they're more active and maintain a healthier lifestyle overall, for example. If you were to change the amount of fat (or any other nutritional component) in your diet while maintaining a similar energy intake, you'd need to change another aspect of the diet as well to make up for the lower fat intake[134] – so two dietary components would need to be modified instead of just one. It's also very difficult to do controlled studies in human beings since we all have different physiological responses to diet and exercise.

Nutritional studies have to be huge and expensive to produce convincing results.

Carbohydrates are the primary energy source for our microbes. The carbohydrates most accessible to them are simple sugars, like sucrose (regular sugar), glucose and fructose (most sugars in fruit, honey and vegetables),[135] since they're easy to break down and use. Too much sugar – especially fructose, which our bodies absorb more slowly than other sugars – provides our bacteria with a huge amount of energy. Excessive sugar leads to an increase in a small number of bacteria, which makes our microbiome less diverse and throws it out of balance.

These features of a poor diet – high in energy, fat, protein and sugars – are typical in Westernised countries. Not only do they contribute to an unhealthy microbiome and whole-body inflammation (which is linked to high rates of chronic inflammatory diseases),[136] they also lead to a lower intake of other essential and beneficial elements, especially fibre.

Our inner microbial ecosystem is a dynamic living community that shapes itself around what we feed it. ('Garbage in, garbage out', as the old computer science saying goes.) Making a few dietary and lifestyle adjustments to help our beneficial bacteria thrive is one way we can improve our health overall.

Intermittent fasting and our gut community

Changing *when* we eat also changes our microbial composition, even if *what* we're eating (in terms of nutrients) stays exactly the same. Waves of digestion and absorption processes happen between meals: over time, this changes both the availability of nutrients to our gut microbes and to our own metabolism.

When we're fasting, the bacteria in our gut have much less access to dietary nutrients compared to the nutrients our own tissues create. The microbes that can forage on compounds we provide (like mucus) are the ones better able to grow.[137] But too much bacterial degradation of the mucus layers that line our gut can also make our gut walls lose their structural integrity and become 'leaky', leaving them open to pathogens that trigger inflammatory immune responses.

While this is a risk with extreme calorie restriction or long periods of fasting, intermittent fasting (an eating pattern that alternates between periods of fasting and eating) seems to have balanced outcomes.[138] This suggests that the outcome depends on how long calories are restricted.

Table 1. Common dietary strategies and their impacts on gut microbial communities

Strategy	Health rationale	Microbial effect
Calorie restriction	Helps weight loss	• Encourages cells to forage for their nutrients (host-forager strategy). • Limits cells from getting their nutrients from food molecules (diet-forager strategy).
Macronutrient distribution	• High-protein diets control appetite and build muscle • Low-carb diets control glycaemic response • No-carb or low-carb carb diets make cells break down our body's fat stores (producing an acid called ketones, which become our body's main energy source)	• Protein versus no protein drives the growth of nitrogen-metabolising bacteria. • Increased fibre selectively stimulates microbes. • Increased fat may select for bile-tolerant microbes, or against bile-sensitive ones.

Strategy	Health rationale	Microbial effect
Intermittent fasting	Promotes metabolic health	• Encourages the use of host-derived nutrients (like urea or mucus). • Makes our fasting metabolism last longer. • Facilitates the growth of microbes which produce layers on cell surfaces (biofilms) that aren't affected by treatments (e.g. antibiotics).
Component quality	Supports healthy metabolism (low-GI carbs)	Slow digestion helps microbes access the nutrient they need.

Dr Clare Bailey's Nutrition Tip #3

Reduce your window for eating to give your gut and the microbes within a chance to recover and do some overnight maintenance. This is known as TRE (Time Restricted Eating): it involves stopping eating by early evening, and not eating or having drinks containing calories until later in the morning. This might mean stopping eating at 6pm and not eating again until breakfast at 8am; that would establish a pattern of 14–10, with a window of 14 hours fasting overnight then eating meals within a 10-hour window. Or you might have a wider window of eating following a 12–12 pattern, perhaps from 7pm to 7am.

Dr Clare Bailey's Nutrition Tip #4

Eating mindfully means paying more attention to what you're eating, savouring the tastes, flavours and textures, and being aware of your food experience and physical cues. You relax and slow down, chew thoroughly, remove distractions and are more able to stop when full. One way to encourage mindful eating is simple: sit at a table and enjoy the company of others. The combined effect of this scenario – as opposed to, for example, sitting in front of the TV or a screen, munching away without thought or appreciation – allows you to take stock of the physical signals that tell your body you're full, allowing you to avoid over-eating. Also, if you're around others, not only will you eat less but it's likely to lift your mood too, and a better mood can, in turn, reduce inflammation.

What would a 'healthy' microbiome look like?

In the same way that human genomes are different for every person (making it challenging to link diseases to specific genetic mutations), our individual microbe communities are different as well, making it difficult to define the characteristics of a 'good' or 'bad' microbiome. So it's not really useful to talk about just *one* human microbiome – instead, we talk about the *many* different human microbiomes.

Scientists usually compare healthy people's gut microbiome to those of patients with specific diseases. If the microbiome composition is different, this implies that the disease is linked to changes in the gut microbiota. But it isn't always easy to define what's a *cause* of the disease, and what's an *effect* of the disease.

And since our individual microbiomes are all different, it's not surprising that the same microbiome treatment or intervention can have different outcomes in different people. A diet that works for one person might not work for another – it could even make the situation worse.[139]

Instead of asking yourself 'what should I eat to get a good microbiome?', a better question might be 'what should I eat to support my *own* microbiome?'. As we'll see in the next chapter, it might help to follow a diet more closely connected to your genetic heritage and dietary ancestry. And food diversity is key.

7

The rise of the modern Western diet

Until around 100 years ago, people were more likely to die from infection than any other disease. Today, non-infectious diseases are also major threats to our health and wellbeing. The World Health Organization recently reported that the top three causes of death globally were stroke, ischaemic heart disease and chronic obstructive pulmonary disease (COPD or emphysema).[140]

Western populations (especially the less privileged members of the population) have had a diet high in processed foods, unhealthy fats and protein for the last 50 years or so. It's no coincidence that since then, despite improvements in health preventatives and treatments, we're getting sick at higher rates – asthma and allergic diseases, for example, are now twice or three times more common than they were. Arthritis cases have gone up by 8% since 1990, and inflammatory bowel diseases have doubled or tripled in the last 20 years.[141]

And in Westernised countries (i.e. Australia, New Zealand, Canada, the US, the UK, Iceland, Norway, Switzerland and most countries of the

European Union) around 30% of the population is now clinically obese, a factor in many inflammatory diseases.

It's now very clear: poor diet and lifestyle can cause chronic disease and lower our life expectancy.[142] Researchers are still working out how this happens so we can stop it.

Diet through the ages: from earliest Africa

Human life began in Africa. Until the end of the Ice Age (11,700 years ago), we all lived as hunter-gatherers, so the human diet depended on local native flora and fauna. Sudden and extreme climate change across Northern Africa at the end of the Ice Age reduced vegetation across the region. Humans migrated out of Africa as vegetation and food resources were lost.[143]

The rise of agriculture

Humans began to farm and develop agriculture around the end of the Ice Age. Farming and agricultural practices spread across the globe from five specific areas: tropical West Africa, the Fertile Crescent across the Middle East, Southern China, Northern Central America and the Orinoco River region in South America. It's been suggested that human migration and the spread of farming practices from these areas happened at the same time, and that local hunter-gatherer populations were overtaken by the migrating farmers' culture and genes.[144] This created the foundation for the modern era's traditional diets – but also narrowed the diversity of our food resources.[145]

But hunter-gatherer practices stayed around in climates where agriculture and farming were unsustainable. In cold/dry climates or unfertile land, it was harder to forage or grow plants, making people dependent on animal products for nutrition. Most environments were fertile, though, and agricultural practices flourished. Warmer climates meant more diverse plant life so people in those areas had a better balance of plant-based foods in their diet. The local flora and fauna defined the traditional diets of different regions.

Let's take a closer look at the traditional diets indigenous to three significant regions of the world: Asia, the Mediterranean and Northwest Europe.

Traditional Asian diets[146]

Green leafy vegetables, legumes, soy foods and whole grains are daily staples of traditional Asian diets, as is rice and fermented products like kimchi and tempeh. Nuts and legumes are the main source of protein, with fish or shellfish eaten about twice a week. Eggs, poultry and healthy cooking oils, like peanut and sesame seed oil, are eaten in moderation. This diet is traditionally low in meat and dairy foods, probably due to the landscape and climate being unsuitable for raising sheep and cattle.

Asia is the world's largest continent, stretching from the eastern Mediterranean to the western Pacific Ocean. Since 770BCE, cooking methods like boiling, steaming, deep-frying, stir-frying and pickling have been used. The establishment of the Silk Road around 114BCE brought ingredients from western regions to Asia – including walnuts, cucumbers, pomegranates, peaches, apricots and cheese.

Thanks to the diverse climate and terrain across this vast region, agricultural practices and diet are different depending on where you are. Different crops dominate different districts throughout Asia, and this has a major influence on the local diet. For example, rice is the dominant crop across Southern Asia (e.g. Vietnam, Pakistan and Sri Lanka), whereas wheat is the dominant crop in countries across the Black Earth Belt (connecting northern Asia to southern Europe), followed by barley and corn.

In Southeast Asian countries like Thailand, Vietnam and the Philippines, rice is a staple and the main crop. Other crops include root vegetables like taro and yam, and fruits like bananas and mangoes. Fish and other sea creatures (including crustaceans and molluscs) are a big part of the diet across east and southeast regions of Asia, especially along coastal regions and in the extensive river deltas. In southwest

Asia, domestic crops include wheat, barley, legumes, cherries, peaches and grapes.

Across northern Asia, foxtail millet, soybeans, wheat and corn are common crops. The vast rivers of northern Asia also offer freshwater fish and other seafood (including crustaceans and sponges) in abundance. The northern grasslands are the original home of burrowing rodents, deer and cattle in Asia. Wild sheep and goats live in the mountains. Animals like horses and yak were used for transportation and for carrying freight, goods or supplies rather than being eaten. Their milk is used to make butter in southern countries like India and Sri Lanka.

The Mediterranean diet[147]

Cereals, vegetables, fruit, yoghurt, cheese, olive oil, nuts, and wine in moderation are staples of the Mediterranean diet. These are eaten daily, along with a weekly intake of fresh fish and legumes, and limited consumption of red meat. The climate and terrain around the Mediterranean Sea shapes this diet.

The Mediterranean region has mild wet winters and hot dry summers. This climate, along with necessary irrigation and agricultural practices, means grains like wheat, barley and rice can be grown. A huge variety of fruits and vegetables are grown in the region too – apples, pears, bananas, figs, date palms, peaches, citrus fruits (especially oranges), potatoes, lettuce, cauliflower and peas, among others.

Fruits and vegetables have been essential to Mediterranean farming and diet since the days of the Roman Empire (27BCE – 476CE). Olive trees are adapted to steep slopes, and their long root systems are suited to survive the long dry summers. Drought-resistant grape vines also grow on the steep slopes. The abundance of olives and grapes is reflected in the use of olive oil and moderate consumption of wine. The Mediterranean Sea provides fish and seafood to supplement the diet, but dry summers make it hard to keep livestock (apart from sheep and goats), so beef is rarely eaten.

Traditional diets of Northwest Europe[148]

Throughout the ages, Northwest Europe has been home to two of the most productive agricultural systems: mixed farming and dairying. (Mixed farming is the use of both crop cultivation and livestock.) Europe can be divided into the dairy belt (the British Isles, Scandinavia and the coastal regions of France and Germany) and the commercial crops and livestock region (central Europe, the Balkans and western Russia).[149]

The major crops during the Roman Empire were oats, barley, wheat and rye, up until the Middle Ages. Then we start to see evidence of peas and lentils being grown but, unlike in the Mediterranean, fruits and vegetables weren't significant. Farmers kept livestock – mostly pigs, since cattle were raised as working animals instead of food. Sheep farming became popular across England, Germany and Norway during the 4th century, which led to cereal production being replaced with dairying.

The introduction of the heavy plough in the 8th–9th centuries and other technological advances meant farmers could work smarter, not harder. Less laborious farming practices lead to more food being produced. The 8th century also saw the production of cattle for meat and milk, and sheep for wool and mutton.

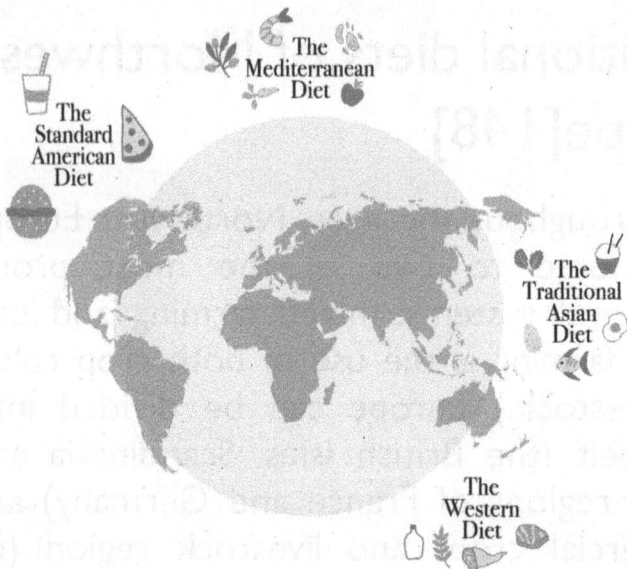

The Mediterranean Diet

The Standard American Diet

The Traditional Asian Diet

The Western Diet

Compared to Asia and the Mediterranean, the cultivation of crops and livestock resulted in a limited variety of foods in the Northwest

European diet. In fact, this basic diet has been described as:

> always the same food and how dreadfully monotonous, no variety, no contrasts. Seldom more than three dishes to a meal, and frequently only two. First, a plain vegetable soup. Second, a meat in slices accompanied by two vegetables, always one white and one green. Third, a dish of bread and cheese or fruit, or on better occasions, both. These Europeans have a singularly uniform approach to gastronomy.[150]

Saving the bounty: food preservation

Finding ways to preserve food has been essential to our survival: food preservation methods like salting, fermentation, smoking and drying have been around for thousands of years.

The Industrial Revolution (1760–1820) sparked an evolution in food processing. New technologies were introduced for mechanically processing farm produce. In the 19th century, processing methods like pasteurisation and canning began to be used.

During the 'second industrial revolution' (1870–1914), scientific breakthroughs saw the importance of nitrogen in plant nutrition, leading to the development of chemical fertilisers which helped stop crop failures and lowered starvation rates.[151]

The 3 stages of modern food processing

The evolution of food processing methods contributed in a big way to shaping dietary patterns throughout the ages.

1. **Primary processing:** when a farming or agricultural product is transformed into something more suitable, palatable or easier and more convenient to eat (e.g. cattle to steak, pasteurising milk)

2. **Secondary processing:** creating food items from individual ingredients (e.g. baking, fermenting, sausages)

3. **Tertiary processing:** preparing ready-to-eat meals (e.g. frozen meals, sandwiches, fast food)

The modern era and the Western diet

Society changed dramatically after the First World War, thanks to the Great Depression and gender roles evolving over that period. This drove the need to be more economical with time and money. Innovative farming practices, food processing and manufacturing met these needs: they paved the way for mass production of food and fast-food restaurants, which spread out first across North America and Western Europe, then the rest of the world.

The demand for fast, tasty, convenient and cheaper food options had a huge influence on Western diets. The Western diet features high levels of fatty and processed meats, unhealthy fats, refined grains, salt, sugar and excess alcohol, while often lacking in fruits, vegetables and dietary fibre.[152] The foods are usually produced by tertiary-level processing (see box entitled "The 3 stages of modern food processing") and contribute to the rise in acute and chronic inflammatory diseases in Western nations.

Western diets: an inflammatory time bomb

Looking back in time at diets that have sustained us across millennia, it becomes abundantly clear that the modern Western diet is out of step with what our bodies need.

Before industrialisation and tertiary food processing methods, our ancestors ate a far wider range of seasonal and locally sourced foods, featuring fresh or fermented ingredients. Meat and fish were caught or farmed in small herds, and not subjected to the chemical cocktails given to factory-farmed animals today. Animal organs high in nutrition were highly prized, foods were cooked in naturally occurring oils with minimal processing (olive oil, lard, butter, ghee) and natural sweeteners like honey were used.

While different cultures' traditional diets can be extremely different depending on the local climate and geographical terrain, what they do have in common is a reliance on minimally processed, nutrient-dense food.

Our bodies evolved with traditional diets over thousands of years. We're genetically programmed from our ancestors and the environment our ancestors survived in.

Their traditional diets are what our bodies function best on – and they're also what our gut microbiome evolved with.

When you look at it this way, it's not surprising the modern Western diet – with its overly processed, chemically loaded packaged foods, heavy in salt, unhealthy fat and sugar, and lacking the fibre and phytonutrients (e.g. antioxidants, vitamins, carbohydrates, amino acids) we need – is linked to so many chronic diseases and poor health outcomes.

Food industrialisation also increased our exposure to chemicals like herbicides, pesticides, hormones and antibiotics that earlier generations weren't exposed to.

This unnatural way of eating is contributing to a too-high baseline inflammatory load and an increase in inflammation-related disease.

If we want our microbiomes to flourish, we'd do well to look to what our ancestors ate and adopt a wide-ranging, diverse diet that's not necessarily focused just on individual macronutrients, but on clean, minimally processed whole foods.

Advances in nutritional science

Thanks to scientific and manufacturing advances, we can now isolate and test individual components of our food. This ability created a 'reductionist' model that links specific nutrients to health and disease.

Reductionism:

Studying only parts of diet instead of looking at it holistically, or single food components rather than food habits.

The early 20th century was an era of vitamin discovery – many of the essential vitamins we know today were identified, and we developed the ability to synthesise them. Vitamin B1 was discovered in 1913 by Casimir Funk. Vitamin C was first isolated in 1932, some 200 years after the discovery that lemons could cure scurvy (which is caused by a vitamin C deficiency). The once-popular food-based strategies to correct nutrient deficiencies were quickly replaced by individual vitamin supplements, launching the billion-dollar modern vitamin industry.

The rate of chronic diseases went up between the 1950s and 1970s, prompting a new focus on the role of dietary fats and sugars in these diseases. The idea that fat was a major contributor to heart disease became widespread. But this belief was based on small studies: it's now understood the reductionist research model doesn't translate well to chronic diseases, being too simplistic to take into account the complex nature of the underlying disease processes involved. The 1970s to 1990s saw a further rise in diet-related chronic diseases.

Today, we've moved to a more holistic view of diet quality and a focus on addressing the massive health burden of chronic diseases. Looking at our nutrition as a whole helps us understand the overall impact of what we eat.

For decades, the reductionist approach dominated dietary research. Its goal is to identify specific components — like fibre, individual nutrients and (more recently) specific plant-based chemicals — that increase or lower the risk of specific diseases.[153] Since the 1990s, many large nutrition studies have provided high-quality data to highlight the limitations of a single-nutrient approach to addressing health issues, and the positive results from using a 'whole of diet' approach as we see in traditional Asian diets or the Mediterranean and Okinawan diets.[154]

Eating for good health: the simple big-picture view

We know that supplementing our diet with single nutrients or phytochemicals (plant-based chemicals) might not have a big impact on the overall burden of disease. Focusing on our overall diet's *quality* by eating whole foods and avoiding processed foods is more likely to help prevent and treat chronic disease long-term.

While our modern lifestyles and environments are dramatically different to those of our ancient ancestors, we're the result of their genetic make-up. Agriculture and animal husbandry – cornerstone practices driving the rise of modern societies – only happened around 10,000 years ago (a mere blip in the evolutionary scheme of things), too recently for our human physiology to adapt to a new heavily processed diet and the 'unnatural' environment of the modern world.

Consequently, in terms of our diet, cultural practices and levels of physical activity, we're living in an evolutionary imbalance with our genetically determined biology. This is thought to be a major contributor to the health issues we face today.[155]

Disease spotlight: How Western diets fuel asthma

As one prime example of how the Western diet can contribute to (or exacerbate) chronic health conditions, let's zoom in more closely on a very common one – asthma.

Asthma is an inflammatory airways disease that affects around 300 million people worldwide.[156] It's more common in Westernised countries like the United States, United Kingdom, Australia and New Zealand. Asthma kills one person a day in Australia.[157]

Asthma is caused by an immune system that over-reacts to triggers like allergens, smoke, viruses and air pollution. In most people, these triggers might cause mild discomfort and symptoms that last for a few days. But for a person with asthma, triggers cause the airways to become inflamed, swollen and twitchy, leading to symptoms like coughing, breathlessness and wheezing. Most alarmingly, people with asthma can experience very sudden, intense flare-ups and have life-threatening asthma attacks.

Asthma has numerous causes. Genetics are important, and if you have a family history of asthma or allergies, you're much more likely to suffer from asthma. As children, boys are more likely to have asthma than girls, but during puberty this switches to women being more likely to have asthma than men. Some people who migrate from a developing country to a Westernised country also develop asthma, which suggests that environmental and dietary factors may be important.

Asthma and obesity

Western diets are likely to play a big role in asthma development and progression. They make inflammation worse by changing the amount and type of nutrients being consumed.[158] Westernised diets contain large amounts of 'discretionary foods' – foods that are high in energy, but have no nutritional value.

Some of the most common examples are convenience or 'fast' foods, cakes, muffins, scones, pastries, wine, beer, soft drinks, sweet biscuits, chocolate and chips/fries. These foods can be eaten occasionally as a treat within a healthy diet, but they introduce extra calories without providing any helpful nutrients, so they are the first foods that should be cut out to avoid weight gain.

Unfortunately, these foods are cheap and convenient; many of us today rely on them. The last Australian Health Survey found 35% of Australian adults' energy intake comes from discretionary foods.[159] No doubt this is driving the obesity epidemic in Australia and worldwide.

Obesity rates have reached epidemic proportions globally, affecting more than 1 billion people.[160] In Australia, over 30% of adults are obese,[161] while in the United States 40% of adults are obese.[162]

Being overweight or obese doubles your risk of having asthma, worsens asthma symptoms and reduces lung function.[163] This is possibly due to the inflammation that develops with obesity.[164] When you gain weight, adipose tissue (fat tissue) can accumulate around your body. As weight gain continues, the cells in fat tissue expand so they can store more and more fat. The more this process continues, the more the cells become stressed and release chemicals into the bloodstream which activate the immune system, causing inflammation that circulates around the entire body.

This inflammation has harmful long-term effects.

Asthma and fat intake

Westernised diets usually contain too much saturated fat. Ingested in excess, these fats cause inflammation because the immune system responds to saturated fat molecules in the same way it responds to bacteria. Immune cells circulate throughout our blood streams, detecting any foreign bodies that may be harmful. These cells have receptors on their surface that detect harmful substances – the same receptors that sense bacteria also sense saturated fat. Immune cells respond to the fat by releasing chemicals to destroy and remove foreign bodies.

So, if you're regularly eating an excess of saturated fat, your immune system is continually activated, causing inflammation to be constantly present throughout your body.

In a study of adults with asthma, a single fast-food meal made airway inflammation worse just four hours later. The meal also made the asthma rescue medication (Ventolin®) less effective, and its effects wear off more quickly.[165] This is a big concern, since asthmatics use their rescue medication for relief during potentially life-threatening asthma attacks, and to stop flare-ups during exercise. This really highlights the importance of keeping fast foods to a minimum if you have asthma.

Asthma and fibre

Fibre intake is also often inadequate in Westernised diets. Our fruit, vegetable and whole grains intake is well below dietary recommendations.

Dietary fibre can be either soluble or insoluble: this determines the fibre's health effects. Insoluble fibre can't be digested and passes through the gastrointestinal tract intact. It's needed for producing faeces and removing solid waste from the bowel. Soluble fibre is digested by bacteria in the large intestine, producing beneficial compounds (e.g. short-chain fatty acids) that reduce inflammation.

Research has also linked fibre intake to lung health. In asthmatic adults, a single dose of soluble fibre reduced airway inflammation after just four hours.[166] In another study, adults with asthma taking soluble fibre supplements twice a day for a week showed an improvement in their asthma symptoms and inflammation in their airways.[167] These studies suggest that poor-quality, low-fibre diets offer less protection against airway inflammation and are likely to make asthma worse.

Asthma and antioxidants

Not having enough fruits, vegetables and whole grains in our diet leads to a low intake of antioxidants (e.g. vitamin C, vitamin E, carotenoids, flavonoids). Antioxidants protect us against 'free radicals' – small, highly reactive molecules that kill bacteria and viruses – but they also damage any cells they come in contact with as a side effect.

Free radicals are constantly produced by the over-active immune cells in the lungs of people with asthma, so their antioxidant defences need to be boosted. You can get antioxidant supplements, but the most effective strategy is to eat more antioxidant-rich foods, especially fruits and vegetables. Whole foods generate more antioxidants during digestion than supplements do. In a seven-day trial, two tomato-based treatments reduced airway inflammation in asthma.[168] In another 14-week study, a diet rich in fruit and vegetables halved the risk of asthma attacks.[169]

A whole-food approach is ideal – more fruits and vegetables in your diet boosts your consumption of multiple antioxidants along with dietary fibre and other plant-based chemicals that together provide a benefit.

Healthy diet and lifestyle the key

This quick snapshot shows how Westernised diets cause inflammation and make asthma worse.

Based on the evidence to date, disease management guidelines now include healthy eating advice for asthma. The advice focuses on achieving and maintaining a healthy weight, eating plenty of fruit and vegetables every day, and eating fewer processed or take-away foods that are high in unhealthy fats and other nasties.[170] These simple strategies can benefit us all.

Diet, genetics and epigenetics

Genetics are a factor in many inflammatory diseases. Except for identical twins, each of us is genetically different and that includes our inflammatory and immune responses.

Our genetic make-up has a major impact on how we process and use the food we eat. For example, some people are genetically unable to taste certain sweeteners and chemicals (e.g. phenylthiocarbamide), changing the way food tastes. Or, to use another example you might be more familiar with, chemicals in toothpaste block sweet receptors on your tongue, which is why orange juice always tastes very bitter once you've brushed your teeth!

Genetics play a major role in obesity, although our microbiome may also have a big effect; animal experiments show obesity can be transferred with faecal transfers.[171] In humans, evidence shows that transferring faecal matter from non-obese people to obese people can improve a person's metabolic function.[172]

Epigenetics

The study of how your environment and other factors can affect the way your genes work without changing your natural DNA sequence.

Epigenetic factors also play a major role in our health. Some studies suggest that up to 60% of how we respond isn't related to our own DNA.[173] Age, pregnancy, what we eat, the environment we're exposed to or what we inhale (e.g. cigarette or bushfire smoke, air pollution), and the infections we get throughout our lives are all factors that induce epigenetic changes. These exposures don't change the actual gene sequence in our DNA, but they can change the way our genes behave. So, things like short-chain fatty acids that are produced by our good gut bacteria don't change the DNA instructions encoded in our cells – but they do change *how* and *which parts* of those instructions are read.

All of this can affect our food and taste preferences. Genetics and epigenetics can change the behaviour of factors (like enzymes and inflammatory cells) that metabolise our food and control nutrient intake. It's the overall impact of these changes that determine the outcome on inflammation, and these changes can be modified by diet.

Food availability also changes our biology over time. Surviving mass starvation events actually improves overall population health substantially and increases life expectancy. In contrast, death rates go up during periods of economic expansion.[174] We now think this paradox happens because, overall, a lower calorie intake is better for us. Globally, for the first time, life expectancy is decreasing as we get richer.

In the same way you inherit your ethnicity from your parents, epigenetic changes also have generational effects. To survive starvation, for example, our bodies prioritise metabolising fats and glucose, but over time, this predisposes us to hyperlipidaemia (excess fat molecules in the blood) and diabetes. In Hawaii and throughout Polynesia, populations were shaped according to who could survive long sea journeys: today, Polynesian babies increase in weight over 20% faster than other babies and grow into strong, fast children and adults. People who live in cold climates tend to have more fat in their diets and larger, leaner bodies that store more fat. Indigenous populations who continue to eat traditional diets high in unprocessed, natural foods are protected from heart disease and hypertension.

Dr Clare Bailey's Nutrition Tip #5

Eat like your great grandparents. Their food was relatively unprocessed and their diet more varied, often more likely to include fermented and pickled foods, fruit, vegetables and whole grains, beans and lentils, as well as some meat or fish. Make sure to steer clear of the ultra-processed Western diet of factory-made products.

Genetic changes that demonstrate the concepts

People with genetic changes in their metabolism, like lactose intolerance and coeliac disease, are proof of the links between diet and health. Interestingly, lactose malabsorption is the norm after weaning, and only people with genetic links to some parts of Africa or Northwestern and Central Europe have the ability to digest lactose after weaning.

Here's some more examples of how genetic variation affects different inflammatory diseases and can be modified by diet.

Iron malabsorption related to • haemochromatosis • liver and heart disease • arthritis • diabetes • vitamin B12 deficiency (anaemia) • coeliac disease	This malabsorption can often be treated with iron infusion or supplements as well as diet modification.
Diabetes	Type I: mostly genetic. Type II: can be helped by switching to a low-sugar diet.
Heart disease	For people with high LDL cholesterol, this can be improved by a lower cholesterol diet.
Hypertension	Reduce dietary salt.
Cancer	Diet modification can help as a preventative and to improve cancer immunotherapy.

Understanding how epigenetic factors can affect our individual genes – and how we respond to particular foods – opens exciting avenues for tailoring our diet to our unique health requirements and preventing inflammatory disease.[175]

As we've seen, the scientific and industrial advances of the modern era set the stage for a highly processed Westernised diet that increases our risk of chronic disease. Going back to a more traditional diet that matches our individual genetics might help reverse the many chronic health issues associated with diet.

8

Minimising inflammation: lifestyle and microbiome approaches

At this point, we know excessive inflammation is often an underlying factor in disease development. In the last 100 years, medical researchers have made giant leaps forward in understanding the intricacies of how our immune system works. We can now prevent and treat many inflammatory diseases, and work on solutions (like vaccines) to make inflammation less severe when it happens.

As always, prevention is better than cure! It helps to avoid some of the lifestyle and environmental factors that cause different diseases (see section entitled "Lifestyle approaches to minimising inflammation"). There are some very effective therapies for these diseases, but the therapies often help ease the symptoms instead of treating the disease – when you stop taking the therapy, you still have the disease. There aren't effective treatments for emphysema, for example, and medicine can only control the symptoms of many other diseases, including multiple sclerosis, asthma, diabetes and neurological conditions. And we still don't have a vaccine for the common cold, tuberculosis or HIV.

Almost every drug-based treatment has issues. Treatments like anti-inflammatories, corticosteroids and anti-histamines are used for a range of diseases: they're non-specific in nature, telling us that some disease mechanisms are common across many diseases. It also tells us that the treatments we're using might not be ideal for some diseases.

We don't have a cure for many chronic inflammatory diseases. But we do know that good nutrition leads to a healthy, balanced gut microbiome, which helps keep the baseline level of inflammation under control. This approach can help protect us against developing inflammatory diseases.

Inflammatory diseases affect more than one organ

A lot of the inflammatory diseases we've discussed aren't single-factor or single-organ diseases, but whole-body diseases that affect one organ or area more than others.

When we're exposed to an infection or another challenge (like smoke or a splinter), our inflammatory and immune cells move from the places they initially grow in, like our bone marrow and spleen. The cells (e.g.

macrophages, neutrophils and mast cells) travel through our blood and lymph systems to the site of the infection, where they keep growing and multiplying to help clear it. If the cells get excessive in number or activity, they can cause damage to other tissues. So, a lot of diseases have multi-morbidities (more than two illnesses in the same person at the same time) that we need to consider.

At a glance

Disease	Multi-morbidities
Asthma, hay fever, eczema and food allergies	All part of the atopic march.
Chronic obstructive pulmonary disease (COPD)	COPD patients are three times more likely to have Crohn's disease. Smoking that causes emphysema is linked to almost all the diseases in this table. COPD, heart disease and stroke usually happen together;[176] underlying inflammation plays a major role in developing blood clots and damaging blood vessels, causing them to burst.
Gut disease	About 50% of people with gut disease have pulmonary inflammation.
Influenza	Having the flu makes you more likely to have secondary bacterial infections.[177]
Kidney disease	Linked to diabetes, psoriasis and vasculitis.
Pneumonia, meningitis, sepsis and middle ear infections	Usually caused by the same bacteria (others also cause sepsis) and are interlinked.
Tuberculosis	Linked to smoking and emphysema.

Lifestyle approaches to minimising inflammation

Modern lifestyles often see us living out of balance with our natural rhythms. As well as our poor diets, we're not getting enough sleep or physical activity, and chronic work-related stress, anxiety and depression are common issues. We live in an environment that encourages poor eating and low levels of exercise and harms our health and wellbeing.

External stressors

Sources of stress around us – anything from traumas to daily issues that affect us, like driving at rush hour in heavy traffic to get to work every day.

Internal stressors

Sources of stress inside us, like fear of public speaking when you have a presentation due.

Stress

Stress, from either external or internal sources, triggers several behavioural or physiological responses to help our bodies stay balanced and functioning properly.

Of all our body systems, stress has the biggest impact on the gut–brain axis (the bidirectional crosstalk between the gut and the brain: or, the way our gut and brain send signals to each other). Stress can affect the muscles in our gastrointestinal (GI) tract, changing the way they move (or stop them from moving at all) – cramping, bloating, diarrhoea or a strong urge to urinate can all result from stress. It can change our gastrointestinal secretions, cause leaky gut and negatively impact our gut microbiome. Stress is a very common cause of irritable bowel syndrome (IBS). Psychological stress can change the pathways in our nervous, endocrine (hormonal) and immune systems to trigger IBS attacks.

Lifestyle changes, like getting better quality sleep or more exercise, can help lower stress and inflammation levels. Stress can also be treated by cognitive behavioural therapy and pharmacological therapies (e.g. antidepressants).

Poor or disrupted sleep

Sleep can affect both the gut–brain axis and inflammation levels. Poor sleep quality has been linked to cancer, type 2 diabetes and Alzheimer's disease. Our immune systems and sleep are linked too; poor sleep can disrupt the gut's natural balance, increasing inflammation by altering gut bacteria and inflammatory protein secretions.

Practising good sleep hygiene is one lifestyle change we can make to improve our sleep quality. Sleep hygiene is related to a person's bedroom environment and sleep routines. Optimising your bedroom environment, having a good sleep schedule and maintaining a healthy pre-sleep routine are all elements of good sleep hygiene.

Dr Clare Bailey's Nutrition Tip #6

Try an early morning walk. Going for a walk at any time of day is good for your heart and lungs, but if you go out first thing in the morning, you will also get the benefit of exposing yourself to lots of bright light, which will help reset your internal clock and set you up for the day ahead. You can also enhance the benefits of your walk by increasing the pace at which you walk. A brisk walk means going at least 100 steps per minute. One way to do that (without the bother of counting) is to choose some music that has 100bpm or more.

Exercise

Exercise is essential for good physical fitness, and good physical fitness is essential for good health. Exercise and physical activity improve our cardiovascular and mental health, metabolic function and skeletal muscle mass, which is linked to living longer. Staying active has been proven to promote the growth of beneficial gut bacteria and good gut health.

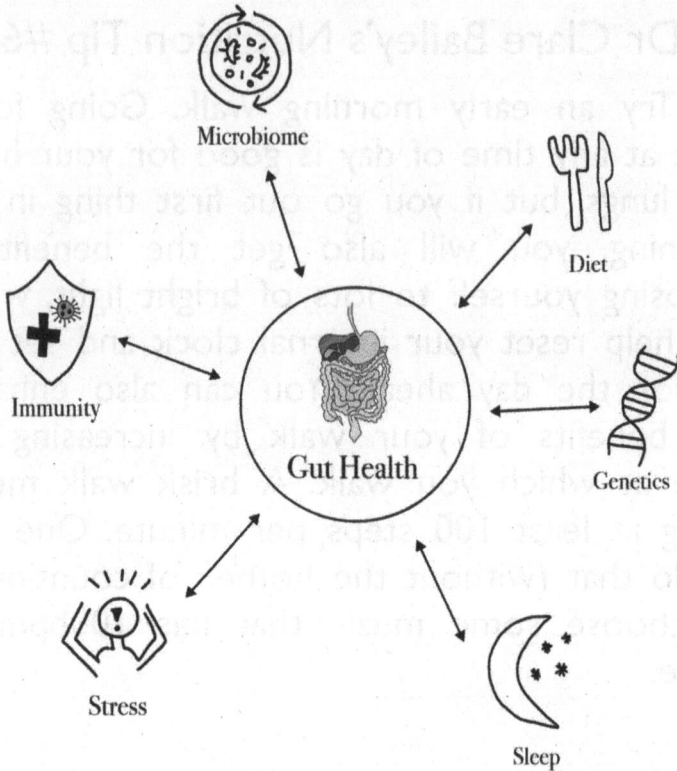

Microbiome

Diet

Immunity

Gut Health

Genetics

Stress

Sleep

Dr Clare Bailey's Nutrition Tip #7

Try to do some resistance exercises most days. These are the sort of exercises where you have to work your muscles against some form of resistance, which could be weights or even your own weight. Push-ups and squats are a very effective form of resistance exercise, though you should check out how to do them properly by going to a gym or finding suitable demonstrations on the internet. The reason it is so important to do some form of resistance exercises is because, after the age of 30, unless you work out, your muscles will start to lose bulk. Having more muscles not only makes you look good, but will keep you mobile and burn calories, even when you're sleeping.

Microbiome-based therapies

Researchers are investigating the potential of microbiome modification to help treat inflammatory diseases.

For years, people have been taking probiotic supplements to boost numbers of friendly gut bacteria. But probiotic supplements don't have much of an effect – likely because they're not based on scientific evidence of how these specific strains actually work in practice. Researchers are still working on identifying more effective (molecularly driven) probiotic strains, ones that work through a scientifically proven mechanism.

One way to modify our microbiome (that doesn't rely on identifying individually critical bacteria) is faecal transplants. If a person has a damaged organ, we can replace it with a transplant – in the same way, if a person has dysbiosis, we can transplant faecal microbiota to give them a 'healthy' microbiome. Faecal transfers are remarkably effective – they take over the existing microbiome and last for months. They've been shown to be 90%

effective in treating some inflammatory bowel diseases.

Faecal transfers are even more effective when people are treated with broad-spectrum antibiotics to wipe out most of the existing microbiome (and potentially bad bacteria) before the transplant, making it easier for the new microbiome to take hold. We may also be able to supplement them with changing the diet to feed the new bacteria.

Hundreds of thousands of these faecal transfers have now been performed throughout the world – there are even biobanks of healthy faeces! There are potential downsides to this treatment, though. In some cases, faecal transplants have actually transferred lethal infectious diseases to the donor, highlighting the need for extensive donor screening. It's also not the most attractive treatment option, when simply modifying our diet could work almost as well.

There's also the potential for microbiomes in other areas around the body (like our lungs and reproductive tract) to be modified, but that's been much less researched.

Recently, a study of the gut microbiome of people with chronic obstructive pulmonary disease (COPD) and healthy controls found 146 bacterial species that were different between the two groups. The levels of some species correlated with reduced lung function in COPD. A set of bacteria and the metabolites they produced were also linked to COPD. This helps us understand how we might be able to modify the microbiome to prevent and treat COPD.

Gut microbiome sequencing is now possible as well, helping us define exactly what's in our gut and what isn't.[178] That includes looking at microbial diversity at the species level, identifying the most abundant species and the metabolites produced by the different bacteria and cells. Some of the pro-inflammatory factors and anti-inflammatory metabolites we assess are listed here.

Anti-inflammatory factors produced by bacteria	Protect against
• short-chain fatty acids vitamins • gamma-aminobutyric acid (GABA)	• infection • inflammation • asthma • obesity • metabolic disease • inflammatory bowel diseases (Crohn's disease, ulcerative colitis, irritable bowel syndrome) • diabetes • hypertension • atherosclerosis and cardiac health • eczema • chronic fatigue • liver disease • colon cancer

Metabolites	Effect
butyrate, proprionate and acetate	suppress inflammation, reduce appetite, metabolise blood glucose and fat, increase serotonin, prevent inflammatory bowel diseases and are an energy source for cells in the gut
succinate	involved in the production of short-chain fatty acids; too much is linked to obesity, diabetes, heart disease
trimethylamine	linked to heart disease and diabetes
ammonia	high levels linked to inflammation and leaky gut
bacterial toxins that promote inflammation	linked to diarrhoea, heart disease, diabetes and obesity
lactate	maintains gut barrier, reduces inflammation and infection; lactic acid bacteria are used as probiotics

Vitamins	Effect
B2 – riboflavin	for metabolising fat, vitamins and amino acid
B7 – biotin	needed for immunity
B9 – folate	for cell repair; low levels are linked to heart disease, stroke and anaemia
B12 – colbalamin	for nervous system and red blood cells
K	helps blood clotting

What does all this tell us?

Despite major advances in medicine, it's obvious that we need a more holistic diet and lifestyle approach to preventing and treating inflammatory diseases – approaches that can be used alone, or along with established drug treatments.

Quitting smoking (or vaping), reducing our intake of alcohol and any drugs, losing weight and improving our diet are factors we can change to improve our whole-body health. Some larger environmental factors are beyond our immediate individual control, though. If we live in cities or close to bushfire areas we'll be exposed to air pollution and bushfire smoke, despite environmental efforts to preserve our natural environment and reduce global warming. We need a stronger commitment from governments and communities to combat climate change.

We know that the higher our baseline inflammation levels are, the more vulnerable we are to disease. Modifying our diet supports a healthy microbiome and lowers our baseline inflammatory load. So what should we eat, and why?

9

What to eat – and why

The word 'diet' usually brings to mind the idea of being 'on a diet': eating nothing but celery, raw carrots and broccoli in an effort to lose weight, for example, or trying to live 'healthier'. But diet is *everything* – all the food and all the drink – you consume every day. That's what we mean when we use the word diet in this book.

Dietary guidelines have been highlighting the importance of good nutrition for years: a whole-food, nutrient-focused, balanced diet helps us stay healthy and live longer. But now we have the science to explain how different food components work at a molecular level instead of just telling us which foods are healthy or not. In other words, we can understand *why* certain foods are healthier than others – and this information can help us decide what to put on our plates. It will be more exciting than you think!

What's the best diet for a healthy microbiome?

To put it simply: there's no single 'best' diet for your gut microbiome. What's important is the *quality* of the food you eat, across your entire diet. Ideally, a well-planned, balanced diet is essential to make sure you're getting the right amount and variety of nutrients.

Dietary guidelines around the world emphasise eating seasonal vegetables, fruits and whole grains while limiting processed foods, especially ones full of unhealthy fats, added sugar and salt. Research also suggests a link between higher levels of toxins derived from gut microbiota and eating more animal fats, sweets and desserts.[179]

In the 'Blue Zones' – geographic regions around the world where people live the longest – a common theme is that their diets are mostly plant-based, with varying consumption of certain animal products. For example, people who live in Okinawa (a Japanese island) and people living around the Mediterranean region are famous for having very long and healthy lifespans. The two population groups have similar dietary habits despite having very different genetics.

Okinawa

Okinawans have the highest life expectancy in the world, and low levels of obesity, diabetes, heart disease and cancer.[180] Globally, Japan has the highest life expectancy overall and is home to most of the people who live past 100 years old.

Okinawans don't have a dietary plan, but a specific way of eating – they eat until they're *satisfied*, rather than full. Their diet features unprocessed whole foods rich in nutrients, fibre and carbohydrates, but low in fat and calories (around 1200 calories per day). They don't eat much meat or dairy – meat is used as a side instead of a main dish. They also eat few grains: the Okinawan diet includes rice, but less than on the Japanese mainland. It's primarily plant-based and rich in yellow vegetables (sweet potato, pumpkin, capsicum), along with tofu, mushrooms, melons and seaweed. These vegetables are high in carotenoids, vitamins, antioxidants and fibre (a common theme in healthy diets), which help to reduce inflammation and maintain healthy immunity.

Okinawans are also very physically and socially active; it's the combination of diet and exercise that contributes to their longevity.

The Mediterranean

There are 21 countries that connect to the Mediterranean Sea, but the Mediterranean diet mainly comes from Greece, Italy, Spain, France and North Africa. It's made up of the foods that people around the region used to eat before processed foods became widespread.[181] These populations have long lifespans with low levels of obesity, diabetes, heart disease and stroke. Like the Okinawans, they follow a particular way of eating rather than a meal plan, and have physically active lifestyles.

The Mediterranean diet is primarily based on fruit and vegetables, nuts, potatoes, whole grains, bread, herbs and spices, with lots of olive oil. Seafood is the main protein source, and chicken, eggs, cheese and yoghurt are sides. The diet is high in vegetables, but low in sugar, grains, animal products, processed meat and trans fats.

Both the Okinawan and Mediterranean eating styles prioritise plant-based whole foods, with minimal processing and unhealthy fats – dietary patterns strongly linked to a long and healthy life with low levels of inflammatory diseases.

The effects of these diets are now being studied at a molecular level. There's a whole research institute, the Okinawa Research Centre for Longevity Science, dedicated to the specifics of how the Okinawan diet is beneficial,[182] giving high confidence that these diets *do* work, and working on explaining *how* they work.[183]

Breaking it all down

As we've seen, our microbiome is intrinsically wired into all aspects of our biology, especially our immune system. It's important to keep in mind that when we're talking about the links between the microbiome and diet, everyone's microbiome is different – your individual microbiome's make-up depends on your age, diet, environment and geographic location. The composition of your unique microbiome affects how useful (or not) different dietary interventions might be for you.

Let's look at how different nutrients and bioactive components in foods affect our gut microbiome, to understand why it's beneficial to prioritise certain kinds of foods in our diets – after all, we eat foods, not individual nutrients!

Antioxidants

Antioxidants are molecules that protect our cells from free radicals (unstable molecules that can harm our cells and may be a factor in heart disease, cancer and other diseases). Increasing our antioxidant intake can be as simple as switching to extra virgin olive oil – 'extra virgin' means it's not processed (the olives were pressed without any heat or chemicals) or adding herbs and spices like celery seeds, cloves and rosemary to your food.

Other sources include tea, dark chocolate (60% cocoa content or higher, and unsweetened) and vegetables like artichokes, broccoli and black beans. Red fruit (e.g. apples, strawberries, cherries) and purple fruit (e.g. grapes, olives, plums) are great sources of antioxidants – the darker the fruit, the more antioxidants it has.

Probiotics and prebiotics

Probiotics are essentially bacteria with health benefits. Fermented foods like yoghurt, kombucha and kefir contain *Lactobacilli,* a bacteria usually found in a healthy microbiome, and are thought of as 'probiotic' (literally, 'pro-life') foods.

Some studies have shown that bacteria such as *Lactobacillus rhamnosus* could help treat peanut allergy,[184] but they are not a miracle food. The specific make-up of our individual gut microbiome will either 'tolerate' or 'accept' the probiotics or they won't.

Prebiotics, better known as dietary fibre, affect our gut microbiome by favouring the growth of specific beneficial bacteria. Science is still unsure how effective prebiotic supplements are, but eating a diet with plenty of fibre-rich foods – in other words, prebiotic foods – will beneficially reshape our gut microbiome. It's dietary fibre that truly feeds our good gut microbes. One consideration is if prebiotics may be more effective if co-administered with the probiotics that metabolise them.

Dr Clare Bailey's Nutrition Tip #8

Probiotics and prebiotics have different functions: the prebiotics act like fertiliser on a lawn to help provide the nutrients for it to grow, while the probiotics are more like the seeds you scatter on the lawn to keep it lush and keep out the weeds. It's a war zone down there in the gut, with the good microbes keeping the bad ones at bay. Feed the good ones and you will reduce inflammation and reap the health benefits.

Dr Clare Bailey's Nutrition Tip #9

Eat fermented foods daily, such as live yoghurts, sourdough bread, pickles, miso, kefir or tempeh. Until recently it was thought that all the bacteria and microbes from these foods would be destroyed by the acid in the stomach, but that has not proven to be the case. These foods are a key part of maintaining gut health. Fermented vegetables such as sauerkraut, or the increasingly popular, spicier Korean version, kimchi, contains both probiotics and prebiotics.

Dietary fibres

Fibre is what we call larger, more complex carbohydrates. Humans don't naturally have the enzymes to break down and digest fibre ourselves – instead, we outsource fibre digestion to our microbes.

Dietary fibre passes through our stomachs and small intestines undigested. When it reaches the colon, it's fermented by our gut bacteria (and other microorganisms like yeast) into smaller components that then use those components as a source of energy. While they're busy fermenting dietary fibre, the bacteria in our gut also generate a range of beneficial anti-inflammatory short-chain fatty acids,[185] which the cells in our body learned to use as humans evolved over millennia.

There's a wide variety of different fibres in unprocessed plant foods (e.g. whole grains, vegetables, legumes, fruits, nuts and seeds),[186] but not all these fibres are equal.

Insoluble fibres (like cellulose and lignin) are found mostly in grains, especially in the hard outer layers. Insoluble fibres bulk up our gut's contents, making us feel full for longer, and help stop us from eating too many microbiome-disrupting proteins, fats and sugars.

While insoluble fibre is essential for gut health, the greatest benefits to the microbiome and reducing inflammation come from two other forms of fibre: soluble fibres and resistant starches.

Soluble fibres include pectin, gums and beta-glucan, and are found in many plant-based foods.

Resistant starches feed the healthy bacteria in our gut. They're found in fruits and vegetables like plantains and potatoes, and legumes like beans, peas, lentils, carob, peanuts and tamarind.

Each type of fibre needs a specialised group of microbes to process it – the most beneficial species being *Faecalibacterium, Bifidobacterium, Lactobacillus, Clostridia, Bacteroides* and *Prevotella* – emphasising the need for plant food diversity in our diet.

Not getting enough fibre in our diet reduces the thickness of the mucus layer that lines our gut. Without fibre, some bacteria species (like *Bacteroides thetaiotaomicron*) resort to breaking down mucus to get the energy they need, leading to 'leaky gut'. This leaves our gut vulnerable to bacterial components (e.g. endotoxins and metabolites) that induce inflammation.

While fibre isn't a complete cure for a poor diet, some research supports the idea that eating over 30 grams daily can help lower your risk of developing chronic diseases like diabetes, heart disease, colon cancer and depression. As a general guide, adults should aim for at least 30 grams of fibre each day.

Top 20 sources of dietary fibre (per serving)

Food	Dietary fibre per serve (g)
Beans (baked, pinto, black, soy)	9.5
Artichoke	6.5
Chickpeas	6.4
Coconut	5.8
Whole wheat bread	5.6
Avocado	5.4
Pear	4.6
Raspberries	4.4
Oats	4.2
Taro	3.8
Peas	3.8
Blackberries	3.8
Jicama	3.7
Lentils	3.6
Apple	3.6
Squash	3.3
Dark chocolate	3.3
Orange	3.1
Almonds	2.8
Hazelnuts	2.7

Honourable mentions, in order: Parsnip, collard greens, banana, green beans, lemon, papaya, mango, sweet potato, macadamia nut, peanut, corn, pistachio, broccoli, fennel, kiwi, water chestnut, nectarine, quinoa, sauerkraut, peach, carrot, date, pasta, olive, pineapple, sugar snap pea, Brussels sprouts, and pecans.

Top 8 sources of resistant starch (per serving)

Food	Starch per serve (g)
Pasta	28.9
Beans (pinto, black, soy)	15.9
Quinoa	13.8
Potato	13
Cashew	7
Banana	5.4
Sweet potato	5.3
Peanut butter	1.5

10 Sources of Insoluble Fibre:

Whole grains

Beans, lentils, legumes

Berries

Turnips and radishes

Green peas

Spinach

Apples

Pears

Avocado

Potatoes and sweet potatoes

Phytochemicals (plant chemicals)

Phytochemicals, also called polyphenols, are chemicals or compounds found exclusively in plant foods. There are more than 5000 different types of phytochemicals[187] – many of which we know very little about. Two of the most studied phytochemicals are *flavonols* (found in dark chocolate, tea, leafy greens and apples) and *anthocyanins* (which give berries their deep red, purple and blue colours). Polyphenols are found across a wide range of plant foods, including herbs and spices (like celery seeds, cloves, rosemary), artichokes, broccoli, blueberries, black beans, olives and extra virgin olive oil.[188]

Around 90% of these polyphenols aren't absorbed in our small intestine, so they travel undigested to our large intestine, where most of our gut microbes live.[189] These microbes use these plant polyphenols as food, and can turn them into potentially beneficial chemicals associated with cancer prevention, as well as cardiovascular and mental health. Studies suggest that eating certain polyphenols found in fruit, seeds, wine and tea might help suppress the potentially disease-causing bacteria species *Clostridium perfringens* and *Clostridium histolyticum.*[190]

Dr Clare Bailey's Nutrition Tip #10

Eat your phytonutrients. Eating a wide variety of plant-based foods helps ensure you get the benefit of a variety of nutrients your body needs; aim to eat at least 30 different plant-based foods a week. More than 25,000 phytonutrients have now been identified – natural compounds that may help to prevent disease and reduce inflammation. These compounds act as antioxidants, which has a fourfold benefit: neutralising harmful free radicals; guarding you from chronic illnesses, including cancer, diabetes and cardiovascular disease; protecting against blood clots; and even improving brain function. You may have heard of the health benefits of resveratrol found in grapes, apples and red wine. The more variety of phytonutrients you consume, the better. By including varied colours, it also makes the food more interesting and appealing, and gets you away from eating a bland beige diet! Further, eating foods of all the colours of the rainbow will give you a better chance of getting the nutrients you need. An apple a day really does keep the doctor away.

Whole grains

Whole grain foods contain nutrients from the grain's bran, germ and endosperm (e.g. wheat, barley, rice and quinoa), in their original proportions. Not only are they rich in fibre, whole grains are also jam-packed with vitamins, minerals and polyphenols.

One cup of whole grain cereal or a half-cup of whole grain pasta constitute one serve, and studies show that increasing our daily whole grain consumption to three serves reduces the risk of coronary heart disease, cardiovascular disease and cancer, and lowers the likelihood of death from all causes – including respiratory diseases, infectious diseases and diabetes.[191]

Protein

Eating too much animal meat combined with not enough plant foods is linked to poor gut health. Unlike animal sources, the protein we get from fruits and vegetables is also full of gut-loving nutrients known to feed a healthy microbiome (fibre, polyphenols, healthy fats and other bioactive compounds).

Having more protein than fibre in our diets is associated with higher levels of gut-derived toxins.[192] Extra protein in our bodies is fermented by our gut bacteria, a process which releases toxins that lead to negative health outcomes (including cardiovascular disease, chronic kidney disease, colon cancer and inflammatory bowel disease).

That's not to say you need to be vegan or vegetarian to have a healthy microbiome – if you're a vegan or vegetarian, you'll still need to make sure to stay away from processed food and make sure your diet is well balanced. For example, whenever you're eating animal-based protein (meats, seafood, milk, yoghurt, cheese, eggs), try pairing it with a variety of healthy plant foods (whole grains, fruits, vegetables, nuts, seeds, spices).

Factory farming

Animal products are a key part of the global diet and often contain micronutrients, particularly vitamins and minerals, that can be hard to get elsewhere. Just as our dietary choices contribute to chronic illness, animals fed an inappropriate diet also become sick and produce less nutritious products. Many animals worldwide are raised in cruel, torturous conditions known as 'factory farms'. These farms can be a vector for infectious disease due to overcrowding and fouled conditions. Poor animal and manure management, meat processing and animal transport can contribute to food contamination and food-borne illness.

Grass-fed vs grain-fed meat

Often the animals we use for food are fed a mixed grain-based diet to fatten them up quickly. These grass-eating animals' digestive systems have not evolved to do this, and switching them to a grain diet can kill the animal if they are not fed antibiotics and switched over gradually. They become bloated and can even suffocate from the pressure on their lungs. Animals raised on grass are much leaner, have five times more omega-3 fats and a much healthier ratio of omega-3 to omega-6s, are lower in the specific saturated fats linked to heart disease, are lower in trans fats and contain a greater variety and abundance of essential vitamins and minerals. What's good for the animal is good for you, too!

Dietary fats

Not all dietary fats are equal. Scientists still aren't sure how the different types specifically affect the gut microbiota, and there is a lot of conflicting information out there about making healthy choices. A simple way to avoid confusion across all food choices is to make sure you prioritise eating real, whole food instead of packaged. Before eating something, ask yourself: 'Is this real food?'

Good fats, bad fats – what's the difference?

Monounsaturated fatty acids

A type of healthy unsaturated fat with only one double bond between carbon molecules. Monounsaturated fats have a number of health benefits: they can help with weight loss, lower risk of heart disease and reduce inflammation.

Omega-6 unsaturated fats

An essential type of polyunsaturated fat that our bodies can't make naturally, so we need to get them from our diet. Omega-6 fatty acids are a source of energy and can protect against heart disease.

Omega-3 fatty acids

A group of anti-inflammatory, essential fatty acids that our bodies don't produce. While we know they are important for brain function and cell growth, some studies also suggest they can protect against breast cancer, depression, ADHD and various inflammatory diseases; however, this is yet to be confirmed.

Polyunsaturated fatty acids

An unsaturated fat with more than one double bond between carbon molecules. These fats are usually liquid at room temperature. Polyunsaturated fats are a healthy fat that can help lower our LDL (bad) cholesterol, which reduces heart disease risk.

Saturated fats

Fatty acid chains that only have single bonds between carbon molecules (unsaturated fats have at least one double bond). Unlike unsaturated fats (like olive oil), saturated fats turn solid at room temperature. Nutrition scientists are still researching whether there's a strong link between these fats and an increased risk of heart disease.

Trans fats

A type of unsaturated fat that comes in both natural and human-made forms. Artificial trans fats increase our risk of heart disease by raising 'bad' cholesterol and lowering 'good' cholesterol levels in our bodies.

Dr Clare Bailey's Nutrition Tip #11

Include seaweed and algae in your diet as it's the best and most sustainable source of much-needed omega-3 oils – after all, that's where most fish get it from. It's also very environmentally friendly as it can be grown in pools of seawater. And if you don't like the taste, you can always get it in capsule form. Two trials led by researcher Dr Pia Winberg, based at the University of Wollongong in Australia, demonstrated that consuming a seaweed extract can be good for your heart as well as your gut.[193] In one double-blind, placebo-controlled trial, 64 patients were randomly allocated to consuming capsules containing either seaweed extract or a placebo. Those who got the seaweed not only saw a 10% improvement in their cholesterol levels, but a 27% reduction in markers of chronic inflammation.

The Mediterranean diet, which contains around 40% fat, has been associated with more diverse gut bacteria and an abundance of microbes that produce more short-chain fatty acids, improving cognitive function and reducing inflammation.[194] The diet emphasises using healthy fats, with olive oil — a rich source of monounsaturated fatty acids — as the diet's main added fat.

The Mediterranean diet also makes use of a number of different monounsaturated fatty acids, like avocado and most nuts, and polyunsaturated fatty acids, like walnuts and oily fish like salmon and sardines, which are high in omega-3 fatty acids.

Western diets have a similar proportion of fat, but with a higher concentration of unhealthy fatty acids. High intakes of total fat are linked to higher levels of *Clostridium bolteae* and *Blautia*, respectively.[195] Both these microbes are related to poorer metabolic outcomes, including insulin resistance. However, these changes don't have to be permanent. In one study, taking daily omega-3 polyunsaturated fatty acids supplements led to reversible changes in the microbiome, including more short-chain fatty acid producers.[196]

Although we are breaking down different foods here, it's actually not very helpful to fixate on individual nutrients. The type and amount of food you eat is more important to a healthy microbiome. A recent six-month human trial looked at how three different diets, with different proportions of carbohydrates to fats, affect the gut microbiota, gut-derived chemicals and inflammation markers. The higher-fat, lower-carbohydrate diet (40% fat mainly from soybean oil, 46% carbohydrate from rice and wheat flour) saw a reduction in short-chain fatty acid producers, along with increases in *Alistipes* and *Bacteroides*, which are linked to glucose metabolism imbalances.[197]

Gluten

Gluten is a protein that occurs naturally in some grains (e.g. wheat, barley, rye). It helps foods maintain their shape, working as a glue that holds food together. Gluten can act as a prebiotic, feeding the good bacteria in our bodies.

It's also a common cause of inflammation. Gluten can damage the gut's mucus barrier, causing leaky gut. Microbes then get into our bloodstream, causing joint inflammation. This becomes chronic inflammation with regular gluten eating. Eating less gluten is likely to help with premature ageing and autoimmune disease.

Food additives and gut health

Food additives are chemicals added to food to increase their shelf life and/or enhance their flavour, texture, or colour.[198] Common additives include preservatives, artificial sweeteners, emulsifiers (which keep fats from clotting together), food colourings and flavour enhancers. The impact of these additives on our gut microbiome hasn't been studied fully, given safety assessments on them were done before we understood the significant role gut microbes play in our health.

Foods with artificial sweeteners have become particularly popular because of their low-calorie content. Sweeteners don't get absorbed and travel through the digestive tract, where they interact with our microbiota directly. Worryingly, animal studies suggest that certain types of sweeteners – especially sucralose, saccharin and aspartame – might change our gut microbiota, drive blood sugar issues and cause liver inflammation.[199] More research is needed to check whether the effects of these food additives are the same in humans.

Alcohol

Having a drink with dinner is common in many Westernised societies, so whenever we talk about diet and health, we also need to talk about alcohol.

As with smoking, alcohol is extremely addictive and linked to a number of diseases. Alcohol also has a high calorie content; wine, for example, contains 250 calories per glass. Unlike smoking, though, alcohol is very much part of the diet enjoyed by the people who live the longest and healthiest lives. Rice wine, or sake, is high in alcohol (about 20%) and is part of the Japanese diet. Wine is also integral to the Mediterranean diet. Provided it's drunk in moderation, there can be some health benefits to alcohol.

Alcohol can improve blood circulation and protect against heart disease.[200] Rice wine contains essential amino acids, vitamins, minerals, antioxidants and lactate-producing bacteria, which can produce additional antioxidants.[201] Red wine has high levels of antioxidants including resveratrol, and increases the levels of good cholesterol (high-density lipoproteins, or HDLs) in your bloodstream. White wine also contains antioxidants including resveratrol, (though much less than red wine) and lowers the risk of heart disease. These effects reduce inflammation and protect against inflammatory and heart diseases. Beer can contain as many antioxidants as wine. It can also contain vitamin B and fibre, both of which lower bad cholesterol levels (low-density lipoprotein, or LDL) and protect against heart and kidney disease.

Still, many of these observations are controversial and not proven – so it's always best to enjoy alcohol in moderation![202]

Bringing it all home: restoring balance

The good news is that healthy eating to support your gut microbiome and general wellbeing really doesn't have to be very hard.

Even just changing a few things can make a big difference.

A balanced diet should contain each of the five main food groups, with an emphasis on fresh, unprocessed food.

What we should eat

When it comes to scientific advice around nutrition, the messages are often confusing, conflicting and always changing. This is why we strongly recommend against focusing on specific macronutrients or ingredients, and instead look across your diet in broad strokes.

Are you eating minimally processed foods wherever possible? Do you seek out a variety of natural, whole foods to eat and enjoy, and enjoy less healthy foods in moderation? Then you are working towards minimising inflammation and improving your gut health.

A good rule of thumb is to imagine your plate or lunch box filled with these portions of the different food groups:

- ½ vegetables and fruit
- ¼ whole grains
- ¼ protein
- and some dairy

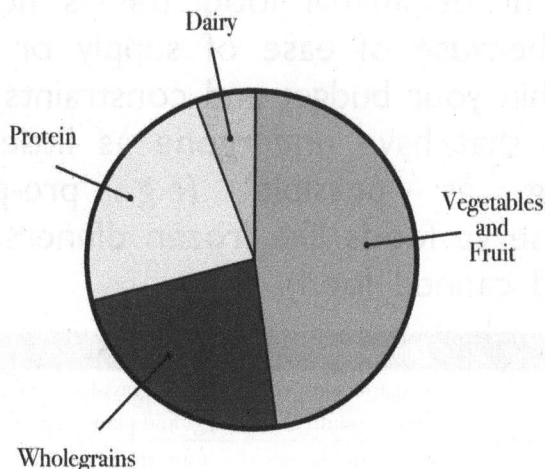

Ideally, we would all be eating a diet made up of fresh, pesticide-, hormone- and antibiotic-free, ethically raised and naturally fed, additive-free organic wholefoods. However, this is not always possible, so keep your focus attainable: a wholefood diet rich with a variety of vegetables, fruit and dietary fibre.

It doesn't matter whether you're eating steaks or beans, nuts or butter, pears or spinach, prawns or salmon – the key is moderation and balance, shifting the focus away from single ingredients and looking at your whole diet to cover your nutritional bases.

Foods to keep on high rotation

While the best foods to prioritise in your diet are any type of organic, free-range, ethically raised plant or animal food, this is not always possible because of ease of supply or cost. So work within your budget and constraints to focus on foods that have undergone as little tertiary processing as possible (e.g. pre-prepared, heat-and-serve foods like frozen dinners, airplane meals and canned food).

Nutrient	Food source
Proteins	Organic meat (high-quality, grass-fed, cooked on the bone), poultry, offal, eggs and plant-based food.
SCFAs and butyrate	Oily fish like salmon, trout, tuna, sardines, mackerel and herring.
Polyphenols	Nuts, seeds, berries, olive oil, brassicas, coffee, tea.
Antioxidants and amino acids	Fruit and vegetables in a range of colours. For irritable bowel disease, it's best to limit sulfur-rich vegetables like cabbage, broccoli and cauliflower.
Prebiotic fibre	Vegetables like artichokes, leeks, onion, garlic are high in inulin prebiotic fibre. Along with prebiotics, seaweed contains vitamins, minerals and omega-3 fatty acids.

Nutrient	Food source
Soluble fibre	Beans, pulses, oats and barley.
Insoluble fibre	Wholemeal bread, bran cereal and seeds.
Bifidobacterium	A small amount of red wine is useful for its *Bifidobacterium* content – bacteria associated with keeping us slim.
Resistant starches	Potatoes, green bananas, legumes, cashews, oats and pasta. When pasta is cooked, cooled and reheated, it increases the amount of resistant starch.

Key concepts to get started

- Focus on **overall diet quality** – avoiding processed foods and consuming whole foods will help prevent and treat chronic disease in the long term.
- A **diverse diet** high in fruits, veggies, whole grains and nuts feeds and promotes a **diverse microbiome.** It also stops us from getting bored with eating the same things!
- Lowering our intake of **high-protein** and **high-fat foods** is an excellent place to start, especially if it means cutting down on processed food. To make sure you're getting enough protein and fat, processed foods can be replaced with moderate amounts of meat as a good source of protein and iron, and oily fish, which provides anti-inflammatory omega-3 fatty acids.

- **Sugars** and **refined carbohydrates** in processed foods can be replaced with complex carbohydrates and fibre from fresh fruit and vegetables, legumes, nuts and whole grains. Of course, you can still enjoy some comfort foods (what nutritionists call 'discretionary foods') now and then – things like cakes, biscuits, pastries, pies and sausages and so on – but try to eat them less often and in very small quantities. A good option is to make your own healthy alternatives, like pizzas with a wholemeal base and some vegetables for the topping.
- Include a **variety of plant-based foods** in your diet for a good supply of micronutrients. If you're pressed for time or on a budget, try using frozen vegetables – they're usually snap-frozen, keeping all the nutrients in them fresh, and have lots of benefits compared to heavily processed snacks. Different cooking styles can affect the nutrient quality of your food, but generally speaking, any plant (even cooked) is better than none.[203]
- **Try not to overeat.** Follow the moderate-intake eating style of Okinawan and Mediterranean diets: eat until you're satisfied, not until you're full.

- Get some **exercise.** Find some way of moving that you enjoy and can work into your day.
- Most importantly – **be consistent!** Just like engine maintenance, it's better to keep things running smoothly all the time rather than fix a problem after there's damage.

The list of healthy ingredients is huge!

Fruits			
acai	dates	key lime	plum
apricot	desert lime	kiwifruit	pomegranate
bananas	dragon fruit	kola nut	quandong
blackcurrant	durian	lemon	star fruit
blood lime	elderberries	lime	strawberries
blood orange	feijoa	lychee	sugarcane
blueberries	finger lime	mango	tamarind
cacao	gooseberries	mangosteen	tangelo
cherries	grapefruit	melon	tangerine
citron	grapes	mulberry	watermelon
clementine	guava	nectarines	winter melon
coconut	honeydew melon	palm fruit	yuzu
coffee	honeysuckle	papaya	*and more!*
cranberries	jackfruit	peach	
cucumber	kaffir lime	persimmon	

Leafy greens			
beet greens	endive	rapini	spinach
bok choy	kohlrabi greens	rocket	swiss chard
brussels sprouts	lettuce	rutabaga	turnip greens
cabbage	microgreens	seaweed	watercress
celery leaves	mustard greens	silverbeet	*and more!*
collard greens	radish greens	sorrel	

Vegetables			
artichoke	eggplant	parsnip	spring onion
broccoli	fennel	pepper (capsicum)	squash
Brussels sprouts	garlic	potato	sweet potato
cabbage	ginger	pumpkin	taro
carob	heart of palm	radicchio	tomato
carrot	horseradish	radish	tubers

Vegetables			
cauliflower	leek	rhubarb	turmeric
celeriac	mushroom	scallions	yams
celery	onion	shallots	zucchini, *and more!*

Legumes			
alfalfa	black-eyed peas	kidney beans	pinto beans
azuki beans	borlotti beans	lentils	runner beans
bean sprouts	broad beans	lima beans	snap peas
beans	chickpeas	mung beans	soybeans
black beans	green beans	peas	split peas, *and more!*

Fermented foods		
apple cider vinegar	miso	sourdough bread
kefir	natto	tempeh
kimchi	pickles	tofu
kombucha	sauerkraut	yoghurt, *and more!*

Seeds and nuts		
acorn	cashew	peanut
almond	chestnut	pistachio
beech	hickory	walnut
Brazil nut	macadamia	*and more!*

Whole grains

barley	noodles	wheat
corn	rice	whole wheat bread
millet	rye	*and more!*

Herbs and spices

anise	coriander	marjoram
basil	daikon	oregano
caraway	dill	parsley
celery seeds	fennel	rosemary
chamomile	lavender	thyme
cloves	lemongrass	*and more!*

Fats and oils

almond oil	coconut oil	olive oil
avocado oil	ghee	palm oil
beef tallow	hemp oil	peanut oil
butter	lard	sesame oil, *and more!*

Animal products

beef	crustaceans	lobster	salmon
brain	deer	milk (reduced fat)	scallops
buffalo	duck	molluscs	sheep
cattle	egg	octopus	snails
caviar	fish	oxen	tuna
cheese	goat	oyster	turkey
chicken	goose	pigeon	urchin
clam	kidney	pork	white fish
crab	lean meat	quail	yoghurt
crickets	liver	rabbit	*and more!*

10

Meal planner

with Fast Ed Halmagyi

Week 1

	BREAKFAST	LUNCH	
MONDAY	Mango & vanilla yoghurt pots with pistachio & mint topper	Cabbage rolls with kale, oat & parmesan filling	
TUESDAY	Brown rice & buckwheat porridge with roasted strawberries & mixed seed sprinkle	Roast chicken, sauerkraut & provolone pan bagnat	
WEDNESDAY	Basil-fried eggs with radicchio & almond toast	Soy & orange glazed tempeh with zoodle salad	
THURSDAY	Simple shakshuka	Chicken pad thai	
FRIDAY	Spiced avocado toast with artichoke-capsicum salsa	Mussel & mixed bean hotpot	
SATURDAY	Wholemeal banana & nutmeg breakfast muffins	Simple sushi with prawns, avocado & seaweed	
SUNDAY	Strawberry puddings with strawberry & dragonfruit salad	Sardine boquerones with grilled sourdough fingers & roasted cabbage salad	

DINNER	DESSERT & SNACKS	
Grass-fed lamb loin chops with whole-wheat kimchi dumplings in pea & garlic hash	Sugar-free rye & berry shortcakes with yoghurt	MONDAY
Rainbow trout 'al cartoccio' with kimchi, broccolini, heart of palm & citrus salsa	Simple vanilla-lemon-ricotta cheesecake with cherry compote	TUESDAY
Linguine 'aglio e olio'	Mixed melon salad with lime & marjoram	WEDNESDAY
Prawn & onion kebabs with grilled corn & bean salad	Easy olive oil chocolate-chunk cookies	THURSDAY
Baharat kofte with golden roasted Brussels sprouts	Date, macadamia & cinnamon rolls	FRIDAY
Slow-cooked lamb shoulder	Homemade cheese sticks	SATURDAY
Roasted mushroom risotto	Whipped vanilla custard with apricots & crisp parmesan-walnut wafers	SUNDAY

Week 2

	BREAKFAST	LUNCH	
MONDAY	Overnight oats with papaya & kiwifruit	Hot smoked trout, pumpkin & fennel salad plate with turmeric & citrus dressing	
TUESDAY	Rye & kefir hotcakes with lemony berries	Seared scallops with carrot purée & herbs	
WEDNESDAY	Coconut & tahini breakfast porridge with spiced banana	Prawn, shallot & snow pea rice paper rolls	
THURSDAY	Herb omelettes with fried tomatoes	Parsley, dill & broad bean falafels with mint-garlic yoghurt	
FRIDAY	Green goddess breakfast smoothie with goat's milk yoghurt	Chicken satay skewers	
SATURDAY	Green eggs, no ham	Spinach & broccolini crepes	
SUNDAY	Frittata with sautéed greens, sweet potato & broccoli	Green linguine with ricotta, lemon & breadcrumbs	
BONUS DAY from Dr Clare Bailey	Scrambled eggs on sourdough toast with smoked salmon & home-made sauerkraut	Easy miso soup with prawns & noodles	

DINNER	DESSERT & SNACKS	
Ciceri e tria: Pugliese pasta & chickpeas	Mocha cake with carob syrup & grape salad	MONDAY
Vegetarian massaman curry of potatoes, celery & tofu	Danish butter biscuits	TUESDAY
Roasted mackerel in green herb crust	Caffè corretto panna cotta with twice-cooked berries	WEDNESDAY
Florentine-style barbecued T-bone with herb butter	Brown butter & raspberry cake	THURSDAY
Braised & chargrilled octopus with garden crudités	Easy lemon tea cake	FRIDAY
Grilled chicken & tomato white corn tostadas	Sugar-free crostoli	SATURDAY
Korean-style braised beef short ribs	Peach & almond tart	SUNDAY
Easy Moroccan chicken tagine	Cheesy parmesan biscuits with rosemary	

BREAKFAST

MANGO & VANILLA YOGHURT POTS WITH PISTACHIO & MINT TOPPER

Preparation time: 5 minutes • Cooking time: nil
Serves: 4

Difficulty: ★★☆☆☆

1 mango, seeded and sliced
2 tablespoons dark honey
2 cups (500g) Greek-style yoghurt
seeds of 1 vanilla bean
1 tablespoon monkfruit syrup [1]
1 cup (125g) toasted muesli
1/4 cup (35g) pistachios, chopped
8 mint sprigs

---

[1] Monkfruit is a fruit native to southern China whose sap produces a taste 250 times sweeter than sugar.

1 Place the mango slices in the bottom of four
   1 cup (250ml) glasses. Drizzle the honey
   around the insides of the glasses.
2 Mix the yoghurt, vanilla seeds and monkfruit
   syrup, then spoon on top, tapping gently to
   flatten.
3 Mix the muesli and pistachios, arrange on
   top, then finish with mint sprigs.

BROWN RICE & BUCKWHEAT PORRIDGE WITH ROASTED STRAWBERRIES & MIXED SEED SPRINKLE

Preparation time: 15 minutes • Cooking time: 30 minutes Serves: 4

Difficulty: ★☆☆☆☆

1 1/2 cups brown rice
1/2 cup (85g) raw buckwheat groats
100g unsalted butter
3 cups (750ml) almond milk
1/2 cup (125ml) honey
finely grated zest and juice of 3 oranges
1 teaspoon vanilla extract
1/4 teaspoon ground nutmeg
2 punnets strawberries, halved

2 tablespoons stevia powder [2]
1 tablespoon almond oil
maple syrup and coconut cream, to serve
1 tablespoon each pepitas, sunflower seeds and poppy seeds

1 Combine the rice and buckwheat in a saucepan with 3 cups (750ml) water and set over a moderate heat. Cook until the liquid has almost been absorbed. Add the butter, milk, honey, orange zest and juice, vanilla and nutmeg and simmer for 15 minutes, until the rice is soft and creamy.
2 Meanwhile, preheat the oven to 140°C. Toss the strawberries, stevia and almond oil in a bowl, then arrange on a lined oven tray. Bake for 20 minutes, until the strawberries are lightly softened and very sweet.
3 Serve the porridge topped with the strawberries, maple syrup, coconut cream and seeds.

---

[2] Stevia powder is the dried leaves of a plant native to Brazil and Paraguay, producing a sensation 300 times sweeter than sugar.

BASIL-FRIED EGGS WITH RADICCHIO & ALMOND TOAST

Preparation time: 15 minutes • Cooking time: 10 minutes Serves: 4

Difficulty: ★★☆☆☆

1/2 cup (125ml) extra virgin olive oil
1 bunch basil, leaves picked
8 eggs
sea salt flakes and freshly ground black pepper
finely grated zest of 1 lemon
4 thick slices sourdough bread
2 tablespoons ABC (almond, Brazil nut and cashew) spread
1 1/2 cups (60g) torn radicchio
2 green shallots, finely sliced
1/4 cup (40g) toasted almonds, finely chopped
75g goat's cheese, crumbled

1   Pour half the olive oil into a large frying pan set over a medium–high heat. Add

three-quarters of the basil leaves and fry until crisp. Add the eggs and reduce the heat to low, frying until sunny side up.

2   Season the eggs with salt and pepper, then scatter with the lemon zest.

3   Meanwhile, drizzle the sourdough with the remaining oil and season with salt. Cook on a hot ribbed griddle for 2 minutes each side, until lightly blackened. Spread with the nut butter.

4   Combine the radicchio, shallots, almonds, goat's cheese and remaining basil in a bowl and mix gently, then set on the toast. Serve with the eggs.

SIMPLE SHAKSHUKA

Preparation time: 15 minutes • Cooking time: 25 minutes Serves: 4

Difficulty: ★★★☆☆

2 brown onions, finely sliced
1 red capsicum, seeded and finely sliced
8 garlic cloves, finely sliced
2 rosemary sprigs, leaves finely chopped
1 teaspoon cumin seeds
1/2 teaspoon coriander seeds, cracked
1/4 cup (60ml) extra virgin olive oil
sea salt flakes and freshly ground black pepper
2x400g cans diced tomatoes
1 tablespoon sweet paprika
2 teaspoons brown sugar
1 teaspoon red wine vinegar
1/2 bunch coriander, chopped
1/2 bunch parsley, very finely chopped
8 eggs
grilled sourdough, to serve

1   Sauté the onions, capsicum, garlic, rosemary and spices in the olive oil in a large skillet set over a moderate heat. Cook for 5 minutes, until the onions are softened, then season generously with salt and pepper.

2   Add the tomatoes, paprika, sugar and vinegar, then simmer for 10 minutes, until the tomatoes are softened. Add half the herbs and stir well, then make small holes with the back of a spoon and crack in the eggs.

3   Cook very gently for 10 minutes, until the eggs are just cooked.

4   Scatter with the remaining herbs and serve with grilled sourdough.

SPICED AVOCADO TOAST WITH ARTICHOKE-CAPSICUM SALSA

Preparation time: 10 minutes • Cooking time: nil
Serves: 4

Difficulty: ★☆☆☆☆

2 avocados
2 garlic cloves, minced
1/2 teaspoon ground cumin
1/2 teaspoon ground coriander
1/2 teaspoon cayenne pepper
1/4 bunch parsley, very finely chopped
finely grated zest and juice of 2 limes
sea salt flakes and freshly ground
white pepper
8 slices rye sourdough
1/2 cup (75g) roasted red capsicum
strips
1/2 cup marinated artichoke hearts,
chopped
2 oranges, peeled and chopped

1 bunch dill, finely chopped
2 tablespoons toasted pine nuts

1 Scoop the flesh from the avocado into a bowl. Crush gently with a fork, then mix in the garlic, spices, parsley, lime zest and juice. Season with salt and pepper.
2 Toast the rye slices.
3 Mix the capsicum slices, artichokes, oranges, dill and pine nuts.
4 Spoon the avocado mixture onto the rye slices, then top with the salsa.

WHOLEMEAL BANANA & NUTMEG BREAKFAST MUFFINS

Preparation time: 10 minutes • Cooking time: 20 minutes Makes: 12

Difficulty: ★★☆☆☆

4 very ripe bananas, plus 1 firm
banana, cut into 4mm rounds
juice of 1 lime
1/2 cup (125ml) extra virgin olive oil
3/4 cup (185ml) maple syrup
1/2 cup (125ml) almond milk
2 eggs
1 teaspoon vanilla extract
2 cups (300g) wholemeal self-raising
flour
1 teaspoon baking powder
1/2 teaspoon ground nutmeg
1 cup (65g) All-Bran cereal
1/4 cup (40g) almond kernels, chopped

1   Preheat the oven to 180°C. Mash the ripe
bananas with a fork, then mix with the lime

juice, olive oil, maple syrup, milk, eggs and vanilla. Add the flour, baking powder and nutmeg, beat until smooth, then fold in the All-Bran.

2   Spoon into 12 muffin moulds (1/2 cup capacity), then top with the firm banana slices and almonds.

3   Bake for 18–20 minutes, until firm to touch. Cool on a wire rack.

STRAWBERRY PUDDINGS WITH STRAWBERRY & DRAGONFRUIT SALAD

Preparation time: 15 minutes + 2 hours chilling
Cooking time: 5 minutes • Serves: 4

Difficulty: ★★★☆☆

3 punnets strawberries, hulled
1/2 cup (125ml) maple syrup
2 teaspoons agar powder
300g silken tofu
2 teaspoons vanilla bean paste
1 can chickpeas
finely grated zest and juice of 1 lime
1 dragon fruit, peeled and diced
8 mint leaves, torn

1 Chop half the strawberries and combine in a small saucepan with the maple syrup. Simmer gently for 5 minutes, until softened.
2 Meanwhile, mix the agar with 2 tablespoons of cold water and set aside for 3 minutes.

3   Mix the agar into the strawberries. Stand for 2 minutes, then purée in a blender until very smooth. Add the tofu and vanilla and purée again.

4   Open the tin of chickpeas and drain 1/2 cup (125ml) of the liquid (the 'aquafaba') into a bowl. Reserve the chickpeas for another use. Whisk the liquid to soft peaks. Add the lime zest and juice, then whisk again until stiff peaks form.

5   Strain the strawberry mixture into a bowl, then add the meringue and fold in gently. Spoon into glasses and refrigerate for 2 hours, until set.

6   Quarter the remaining strawberries and mix with the dragon fruit and mint. Serve with the strawberry puddings.

OVERNIGHT OATS WITH PAPAYA & KIWIFRUIT

Preparation time: 5 minutes + overnight soaking
Cooking time: nil • Serves: 4

Difficulty: ★☆☆☆☆

1/2 cup (50g) rolled oats
1/4 cup (40g) currants
1 tablespoon chia seeds
1 teaspoon ground cinnamon
1 cup (250ml) almond milk
1/2 cup (125ml) apple juice
1/4 cup (60ml) honey
1 teaspoon vanilla extract
1 1/2 cups (270g) papaya, peeled and diced
2 kiwifruit, peeled and finely diced
12 mint leaves, torn
honey and toasted almonds, to serve

1   Combine the oats, currants, chia seeds, cinnamon, almond milk, apple juice, honey

and vanilla in a bowl and mix well. Refrigerate overnight.

2 Gently mix together the papaya, kiwifruit and mint. Spoon the oats into glasses, top with the papaya salad, then serve with honey and toasted almonds.

RYE & KEFIR HOTCAKES WITH LEMONY BERRIES

Preparation time: 15 minutes • Cooking time: 20 minutes Serves: 4

Difficulty: ★★☆☆☆

1 cup (120g) rye flour
1/2 cup (50g) almond meal
2 teaspoons baking powder
2 tablespoons stevia powder
3 eggs, separated
1 teaspoon almond essence
1 cup (250ml) plain milk kefir
1/2 teaspoon cream of tartar
cooking oil spray
1/2 cup (125ml) monkfruit syrup
finely grated zest of 2 lemons
3 cups (375g) frozen berries
Greek-style yoghurt and ground cinnamon, to serve

1   Combine the flour, almond meal, baking powder and stevia in a bowl and mix well. Whisk the egg yolks, almond essence and

kefir in a second bowl, then add to the dry mixture, stirring until smooth.

2   Whisk the egg whites and cream of tartar to soft peaks, then fold into the batter.

3   Set a large frying pan sprayed with cooking oil over a moderate heat. Cook the batter in 1/2 cup (125ml) amounts for 2 minutes on each side, to make 12 hotcakes.

4   Meanwhile, heat the monkfruit syrup and lemon zest in a medium saucepan until boiling. Add the berries, then remove from the heat.

5   Drain the liquid into a second saucepan. Boil for a few minutes until beginning to thicken, then add back to the berries.

6   Serve the hotcakes with the berries, yoghurt and cinnamon.

COCONUT & TAHINI BREAKFAST PORRIDGE WITH SPICED BANANA

Preparation time: 10 minutes • Cooking time: 35 minutes Serves: 4

Difficulty: ★★☆☆☆

1/2 cup (100g) quinoa
1 cup (100g) rolled oats
2 1/2 cups (625ml) coconut water
2x400ml cans coconut milk
1/2 cup (125ml) monkfruit syrup
finely grated zest of 2 limes
cooking oil spray
4 bananas, sliced 1cm thick
1/2 cup (125ml) honey
1/2 teaspoon ground cardamom
1/2 teaspoon ground ginger
1/2 teaspoon ground cinnamon
1 cup (65g) shredded coconut, toasted
1/2 cup (135g) tahini

1   Put the quinoa in a sieve and wash under cold water until the water runs clear. Mix

with the oats, coconut water, coconut milk, monkfruit syrup and lime zest in a medium saucepan and set over a moderate heat. Simmer for 20 minutes, until slightly thickened.

2 Spray a large non-stick frying pan with cooking oil, then fry the banana slices for I minute, until lightly blackened. Add the honey and spices, then cook until the syrup thickens.

3 Spoon the porridge into bowls, then top with the bananas, coconut and tahini.

HERB OMELETTES WITH FRIED TOMATOES

Preparation time: 10 minutes • Cooking time: 20 minutes Serves: 4

Difficulty: ★★★☆☆

1/4 cup (60ml) extra virgin olive oil
6 small tomatoes, hulled and halved
4 garlic cloves, minced
2 French shallots, very finely sliced
2 long red chillies, seeded and very finely diced
sea salt flakes and freshly ground white pepper
12 eggs
2 tablespoons finely chopped herbs (chives, parsley, tarragon, chervil)
100g unsalted butter

1　Pour 1 tablespoon of the olive oil into a large non-stick frying pan set over a moderate heat. Add the tomatoes face down and cook for 5 minutes. Flip the tomatoes over and scatter with the garlic, shallots and chillies. Season generously with salt and pepper, cook for 2 minutes, then flip again and set aside.

2   Whisk the eggs until smooth, then strain through a fine sieve. Season with salt and pepper, then mix in half the herbs.

3   Put one-quarter of the butter in a 20cm non-stick frying pan set over a moderate heat. Once sizzling, add one-quarter of the egg mixture. Cook, scraping the bottom constantly with a heatproof spatula, until the mixture is just beginning to set.

4   Flip the sides over, then invert onto a plate. Sprinkle with more herbs and serve with some fried tomatoes.

5   Repeat to make another three omelettes.

GREEN GODDESS BREAKFAST SMOOTHIE WITH GOAT'S MILK YOGHURT

Preparation time: 5 minutes • Cooking time: nil
Serves: 4

Difficulty: ★☆☆☆☆

2 ripe bananas, peeled
4 kiwifruit, peeled
I green apple, cored
I Lebanese cucumber, seeded
4 cups (200g) baby spinach leaves
1/2 bunch mint
2 teaspoons vitamin C powder
3 cups (750g) goat's milk yoghurt
3/4 cup (185ml) monkfruit syrup
ice cubes

I   Combine the fruit, cucumber, spinach, mint, vitamin C, yoghurt and monkfruit syrup in a blender and purée until very smooth.

2 Add the ice, then blitz until the ice is crushed.

GREEN EGGS, NO HAM

Preparation time: 10 minutes • Cooking time: 10 minutes Serves: 4

Difficulty: ★★☆☆☆

1 bunch parsley, leaves picked
1/2 bunch mint, leaves picked
1/2 bunch tarragon, leaves picked
4 garlic cloves, peeled
2 tablespoons pine nuts, toasted
2 teaspoons capers
1/4 cup (25g) finely grated pecorino cheese
1/4 teaspoon chilli flakes
1/2 cup (125ml) extra virgin olive oil
sea salt flakes and freshly ground black pepper
8 eggs
chargrilled ciabatta and labne, to serve

1   Combine the herbs, garlic, pine nuts, capers, pecorino, chilli and olive oil in a food processor and blitz until a paste forms. Season with salt and pepper. Set aside.

2   Bring a wide pan of salted water to a bare simmer. Crack the eggs into glasses, then gently lower each into the water, tipping out the eggs. Cook for 4 minutes, until just firm. Scoop out and pat dry with paper towel.

3   Serve on chargrilled ciabatta spread with labne, topped with the herb sauce.

FRITTATA WITH SAUTÉED GREENS, SWEET POTATO & BROCCOLI

Preparation time: 20 minutes • Cooking time: 1 hour Serves: 4–6

Difficulty: ★★★☆☆

2 cups sweet potato, peeled
1/2 cup (125ml) extra virgin olive oil
sea salt flakes and freshly ground
black pepper
2 teaspoons honey
2 heads of broccoli, cut into florets
1 red onion, finely sliced
4 garlic cloves, minced
1/2 bunch sage leaves, finely sliced
2 bunches English spinach, roughly
chopped
12 eggs
150ml cream
cooking oil spray

chopped walnuts, lemon wedges, herb salad and rye toast, to serve

1 Preheat the oven to 180°C.

2 Slice the sweet potato into 1cm sticks, then toss with 2 tablespoons of the olive oil and season with salt and pepper. Arrange on a lined oven tray and bake for 30 minutes, then drizzle with honey and bake for a further 10 minutes.

3 Meanwhile, toss the broccoli in 2 tablespoons of extra virgin olive oil and season with salt. Bake on a lined oven tray for 30 minutes, until lightly blackened.

4 Pour the remaining oil into a medium frying pan. Sauté the onion, garlic and sage over a moderate heat for 5 minutes, then mix in the spinach and cook gently until wilted.

5 Whisk the eggs and cream in a bowl and season lightly with salt and pepper. Set a 22cm non-stick pan over a moderate heat and spray with cooking oil. Pour in the egg mixture, then add the sweet potato and sautéed spinach mixture. Cook very gently until the eggs are just cooked.

6 Slide onto a serving platter and top with the broccoli and walnuts. Serve with lemon wedges, a herb salad and rye toast.

LUNCH

CABBAGE ROLLS WITH KALE, OAT & PARMESAN FILLING

Preparation time: 20 minutes • Cooking time: 1 hour 20 minutes Serves: 4

Difficulty: ★★★☆☆

1 head of green cabbage
1 brown onion, sliced
6 garlic cloves, minced
1/2 bunch thyme, leaves picked
2 tablespoons extra virgin olive oil
1 bunch Tuscan kale, torn
1 1/2 cups (150g) rolled oats
1 cup (100g) finely grated parmesan cheese
500ml tomato passata
1 litre (4 cups) chicken stock
1 tablespoon honey
sea salt flakes and freshly ground black pepper

herb salad and sour cream, to serve

1   Preheat the oven to 160°C. Use a small sharp knife to remove 12 outer leaves of the cabbage, then cut out the thick central ribs. Blanch in boiling water until softened, then refresh under cold running water.
2   Sauté the onion, garlic and thyme in the olive oil over a moderate heat for 5 minutes, until softened, then add the kale and cook until wilted. Mix in the oats and cheese. Arrange the cabbage leaves on a workbench, then spoon the kale mixture onto the near edges. Fold in the sides, then roll up.
3   Put the rolls in an ovenproof dish, leaving some room to expand, then top with the passata, stock and honey. Season with salt and pepper, then cover with foil and bake for 1 hour.
4   Serve with herb salad and sour cream.

ROAST CHICKEN, SAUERKRAUT & PROVOLONE PAN BAGNAT

Preparation time: 5 minutes + 30 minutes resting
Cooking time: 10 minutes • Serves: 4

Difficulty: ★★☆☆☆

2 cups (300g) shredded roast chicken
1/2 cup (125g) aioli [3]
1 bunch chives, very finely snipped
4 ciabatta rolls, split
2 tablespoons unsalted butter, at room temperature
1 1/2 cups (225g) red sauerkraut
120g provolone cheese, finely sliced
1/2 bunch basil, leaves picked
1 cup (100g) grilled eggplant slices
baby salad leaves, to serve

---

[3] If you can find it, truffle aioli transforms this dish from incredible to unforgettable.

1   Mix the chicken, aioli and chives in a bowl. Spread the ciabatta rolls with the butter, then top the bases with the sauerkraut, chicken, cheese, basil and eggplant. Put the ciabatta lids on top.

2   Arrange the rolls on a tray, then top with a second tray and weigh down with at least 5kg (a pot of water is good) for 30 minutes.

3   Cook in a hot sandwich press for 10 minutes, until deep golden and crisp. Serve with baby salad leaves.

SOY & ORANGE GLAZED TEMPEH WITH ZOODLE SALAD

Preparation time: 20 minutes • Cooking time: 10 minutes Serves: 4

Difficulty: ★★☆☆☆

4 medium zucchini
2 carrots, peeled
1/4 head of red cabbage, shredded
1/2 cup (60g) bean shoots
1/2 cup (70g) roasted peanuts, crushed
1/2 bunch coriander, leaves picked
1/4 bunch mint, leaves picked
1/2 cup (125ml) light soy sauce
finely grated zest and juice of 2 oranges
3 tablespoons palm sugar, grated
4cm piece of fresh ginger, finely grated
4cm piece of fresh turmeric, minced
4 garlic cloves, minced
1 lemongrass stem, pale part finely chopped

1 tablespoon sesame oil
600g tempeh, in 1cm slices
1/4 cup (60ml) sesame Japanese
mayonnaise

1   Use a spiraliser to shred the zucchini and carrots into noodles. Combine in a bowl with the cabbage, bean shoots, peanuts and herbs, mixing well.
2   Mix the soy sauce, orange zest and juice, palm sugar, ginger, turmeric, ginger, garlic and lemongrass. Set aside.
3   Pour the sesame oil into a large non-stick pan over a high heat. Fry the tempeh for a few minutes until well-browned on both sides, then remove from the pan.
4   Pour the soy sauce mixture into the pan and cook until thickened, then toss the tempeh through. Serve on top of the salad, drizzled with the mayonnaise.

CHICKEN PAD THAI

Preparation time: 15 minutes • Cooking time: 20 minutes Serves: 4

Difficulty: ★★★☆☆

2 chicken breast fillets
180g dried wide rice stick noodles
1/4 cup (60ml) canola oil
2 tablespoons fish sauce
2 tablespoons honey
2 tablespoons tamarind paste
1 tablespoon rice vinegar
1 tablespoon light soy sauce
2 teaspoons chilli flakes
4 green shallots, finely sliced
6cm piece of fresh ginger, cut into fine batons
6 garlic cloves, minced
2 cups (150g) finely shredded wombok
4 eggs, beaten
1 cup (100g) mung bean sprouts
1/2 cup (70g) roasted peanuts
1/2 bunch coriander, leaves picked
lime wedges, to serve

1   Place the chicken breasts in a saucepan of cold water and set over a moderate heat. Simmer for 15 minutes, until firm, then drain and set aside to cool. Shred finely.

2   Meanwhile, cover the noodles with boiling water and stand for 15 minutes, then drain well and toss with 1 tablespoon of the canola oil.

3   Combine the fish sauce, honey, tamarind, vinegar, soy sauce and chilli in a bowl. Set aside.

4   Sauté the shallots, ginger, garlic and wombok in the remaining oil in a wok over a high heat. Add the eggs and mix well until scrambled.

5   Mix in the chicken, noodles, sprouts, peanuts and sauce, then simmer for a few minutes, until thickened. Add the coriander, then serve with lime wedges.

MUSSEL & MIXED BEAN HOTPOT

Preparation time: 15 minutes • Cooking time: 15 minutes Serves: 4

Difficulty: ★★★☆☆

2 leeks, pale parts finely sliced
2 celery stalks, finely diced
6 garlic cloves, minced
1/2 bunch thyme, leaves picked
1/4 cup (60ml) extra virgin olive oil
2kg mussels, scrubbed and debearded
4 ripe tomatoes, seeded and diced
4 fresh bay leaves
4 juniper berries
1/2 cup (125ml) dry sherry
2 cups (500ml) fish stock
1 tablespoon fish sauce
2x400g cans mixed beans, drained
3 cups (150g) baby spinach leaves
2 bunches chives, snipped

1   Sauté the leeks, celery, garlic and thyme in half the olive oil in a large lidded saucepan

for 5 minutes, until softened. Remove and set aside.

2 Pour the remaining oil into the saucepan, then add the mussels, tomatoes, bay leaves and juniper berries. Cook with the lid on for 2 minutes, then add the sherry, cover and cook for another 2 minutes. Add the stock, fish sauce and beans. Cook, uncovered, for 5 minutes, until all the mussel shells have opened.

3 Mix in the spinach and chives, then serve.

SIMPLE SUSHI WITH PRAWNS, AVOCADO & SEAWEED

Preparation time: 15 minutes + 10 minutes
standing Cooking time: 20 minutes • Serves: 4

Difficulty: ★★★☆☆

2 cups (420g) sushi rice
1/4 cup (60ml) rice wine vinegar
2 tablespoons monkfruit sweetener
1 teaspoon sea salt flakes
6 nori seaweed sheets
1/4 cup (60ml) Japanese mayonnaise
12 large cooked tiger prawns, peeled,
deveined and halved lengthways
1 avocado, flesh cut into fine wedges
1/2 cup (50g) seaweed salad
soy sauce, lemon juice, pickled ginger
and wasabi, to serve

1   Put the rice in a fine sieve and rinse under
    cold running water until the water runs clear.
    Transfer the rice to a medium saucepan with
    3 cups (750ml) cold water. Set over a

moderate heat and cook until craters appear. Turn the heat to low, cook for 3 minutes, then put the lid on and turn the heat off. Stand for 10 minutes.

2   Scrape the rice gently with a fork. Add the vinegar, monkfruit sweetener and salt, then stir gently.

3   Working with one seaweed sheet at a time, spread the rice over, leaving a 4cm margin at the far edge, then top with some mayonnaise, prawns, avocado and seaweed salad. Lightly moisten the far edge of the sheet, then roll up tightly using a sushi mat.

4   Slice the sushi logs with a sharp, slightly damp knife. Serve with a mixture of soy sauce, lemon juice, ginger and wasabi.

SARDINE BOQUERONES WITH GRILLED SOURDOUGH FINGERS & ROASTED CABBAGE SALAD

Preparation time: 30 minutes + overnight marinating Cooking time: 1 hour 10 minutes • Serves: 4–6

Difficulty: ★★★☆☆

500g fresh sardine fillets
finely grated zest and juice of 2 oranges
4 juniper berries, crushed
1/4 cup (60ml) apple cider vinegar
2 tablespoons sea salt flakes
1 tablespoon raw sugar
1/2 head of cabbage
3/4 cup (185ml) extra virgin olive oil
sea salt flakes and freshly ground black pepper
2 whole garlic bulbs

4 radishes, finely sliced
I bunch parsley, leaves picked
4 slices sourdough bread

I   Arrange the sardine fillets in a single layer in a glass dish. Mix the orange zest and juice, juniper berries, vinegar, salt flakes and sugar, then pour over the sardines. Cover and refrigerate overnight.

2   Preheat the oven to 200°C. Slice the cabbage into quarters, toss with half the olive oil and season generously with salt and pepper. Arrange on a baking dish. Wrap each garlic bulb in foil and arrange alongside. Roast for I hour, until the cabbage is beginning to blacken.

3   Tear the cabbage into pieces, then squeeze the roasted garlic on top, discarding the skin. Add the radishes and parsley, drizzle with the pan roasting juices, then toss gently.

4   Drizzle the bread with the remaining oil and season generously with salt and pepper. Cook on a hot ribbed grill until lightly blackened. Cut into fingers, then serve with the sardines and cabbage salad.

HOT SMOKED TROUT, PUMPKIN & FENNEL SALAD PLATE WITH TURMERIC & CITRUS DRESSING

Preparation time: 15 minutes • Cooking time: nil
Serves: 4

Difficulty: ★★☆☆☆

2 cups pumpkin
2 red apples
1 fennel bulb
1 red onion, peeled
4 radishes
1/2 cup (50g) pecans, roughly chopped
1/4 cup (40g) pepitas
1 bunch parsley, leaves picked
250g hot smoked trout, flaked
2 oranges, peeled and diced
2 limes, peeled and diced
1 lemon, peeled and diced
1/4 cup (60ml) extra virgin olive oil

5cm piece of fresh turmeric, finely grated
2 garlic cloves, minced
sea salt flakes and freshly ground black pepper

1   Shave the pumpkin, apples, fennel, onion and radishes as finely as possible using a mandoline, then toss lightly in a bowl. Mix in the pecans, pepitas and parsley. Add the trout, then mix one final time.
2   Combine the citrus pieces, olive oil, turmeric and garlic, season with salt and pepper, then whisk well. Drizzle over the salad.

SEARED SCALLOPS WITH CARROT PURÉE & HERBS

Preparation time: 15 minutes + 1 hour draining
Cooking time: 30 minutes • Serves: 4

Difficulty: ★★★☆☆

1kg carrots, peeled and chopped
2 cups (500ml) apple juice
1/2 cup (125ml) extra virgin olive oil
sea salt flakes and freshly ground
black pepper
20 scallops, roe off
cooking oil spray
1 tablespoon salmon roe
2 tablespoons goat's milk yoghurt
2 tablespoons each chopped parsley,
dill, tarragon and chives

1 Steam the carrots until very tender. Transfer to a blender with the apple juice and olive oil. Purée until very smooth, season with salt and pepper, then hang in a muslin bag over a bowl or sink for 1 hour.

2 Sprinkle the scallops with cooking oil spray. In batches, cook them in a non-stick frying pan over a high heat for 1 minute each side, until golden. Season lightly with salt.

3 Spread the carrot purée on plates. Top with the scallops, salmon roe, yoghurt and herbs.

PRAWN, SHALLOT & SNOW PEA RICE PAPER ROLLS

Preparation time: 20 minutes • Cooking time: nil
Makes: 12

Difficulty: ★★★☆☆

120g dried rice vermicelli noodles
12 rice paper sheets
18 cooked prawns, peeled and deveined, then halved lengthways
1/4 bunch coriander, leaves picked
1/4 bunch mint, leaves picked
2 carrots, peeled and grated
4 green shallots, cut into 15cm lengths
12 snow peas, finely sliced
1/2 cup (125ml) oyster sauce
1/4 cup (60ml) hoisin sauce
1 tablespoon fish sauce
1 tablespoon sambal oelek
2 tablespoons honey
1 garlic clove, minced

1 Put the noodles in a bowl and cover with boiling water. Stand for 3 minutes, then drain well. Working one at a time, dip the rice paper sheets into cold water, shake off the excess, then arrange on a lightly moistened board.

2 Place three prawn halves and some herb leaves in a line in the centre, then top with some carrot, shallot, snow peas and noodles, with the shallots sticking out one end. Fold the end of the sheet over, then one side, then roll up towards the other side. Repeat with the remaining rice paper and ingredients.

3 Mix the oyster, hoisin and fish sauces with the sambal, honey and garlic, then serve with the rice paper rolls.

PARSLEY, DILL & BROAD BEAN FALAFELS WITH MINT-GARLIC YOGHURT

Preparation time: 20 minutes + overnight soaking
Cooking time: 10 minutes • Serves: 4

Difficulty: ★★★☆☆

500g dried broad beans
1/4 cup (30g) chickpea flour
1 teaspoon bicarbonate of soda
2 teaspoons ground cumin
2 teaspoons ground coriander
1 teaspoon ground cinnamon
1/2 teaspoon cayenne pepper
1/2 leek, finely chopped
4 green shallots, finely sliced
1 bunch coriander, finely chopped
1/2 bunch parsley, finely chopped
1/2 bunch dill, finely chopped
1 bunch mint, finely chopped
6 garlic cloves, minced

**sea salt flakes and freshly ground
black pepper
1/2 cup (75g) sesame seeds
vegetable oil, for deep-frying
1 1/2 cups (375g) Greek-style yoghurt
finely grated zest and juice of 1 lemon**

1 Cover the broad beans with warm water and soak for 4 hours. Drain, cover again with water, then soak overnight.

2 Drain the broad beans, then blitz in a food processor until a fine paste forms. Add the chickpea flour, bicarbonate of soda, spices, leek, shallots, coriander, parsley and dill. Add half the mint and garlic, then blitz until smooth. Season generously with salt and pepper.

3 Form into 20 balls and roll into football shapes. Coat with the sesame seeds, then fry in batches until golden. Drain on paper towel.

4 Mix the yoghurt with the lemon zest and juice and remaining mint and garlic, then serve with the falafels.

CHICKEN SATAY SKEWERS

Preparation time: 15 minutes + 10 minutes marinating Cooking time: 15 minutes • Serves: 4

Difficulty: ★★★☆☆

800g chicken thigh fillets, sliced into strips
1/2 cup (125ml) honey
2 tablespoons curry powder
1 cup (250g) red curry paste
sea salt flakes and freshly ground black pepper
1 cup (260g) crunchy peanut butter
1/4 cup (60ml) light soy sauce
finely grated zest and juice of 4 limes
1 cup (250ml) coconut water
1/2 cup (125ml) coconut cream
chopped peanuts, lime wedges, coconut cream, coriander, chilli, toasted coconut and Thai basil, to serve

1   Combine the chicken thighs in a bowl with the honey, curry powder and half the curry

paste. Season generously with salt and pepper. Set aside for 10 minutes.

2   Meanwhile, soak 12 bamboo skewers in water, so they don't scorch on the barbecue.

3   Put the remaining curry paste in a medium saucepan with the peanut butter, soy sauce, lime zest and juice, coconut water and coconut cream. Simmer gently for 5 minutes, stirring well, until thickened. Season with salt and pepper.

4   Thread the chicken onto the bamboo skewers, then cook over a moderate barbecue grill for 5 minutes, turning regularly, until firm to touch.

5   Serve with the satay sauce, chopped peanuts, lime wedges, coconut cream, coriander, chilli, toasted coconut and Thai basil.

SPINACH & BROCCOLINI CREPES

Preparation time: 25 minutes + I hour resting
Cooking time: 25 minutes • Serves: 4

Difficulty: ★★☆☆☆

I cup (150g) plain flour
2 cups (500ml) milk
3 eggs
sea salt flakes and freshly ground
black pepper
cooking oil spray
8 broccolini florets (with stalks)
2 tablespoons extra virgin olive oil
I cup (220g) hummus
200g sour cream
2 cups (100g) baby spinach leaves
I green chilli, seeded and finely sliced
soy bean and asparagus salad, to serve

I   Whisk the flour, milk and eggs in a bowl and season with salt. Strain through a fine sieve, then set aside for I hour.

2   Set a 20cm crepe pan sprayed with cooking oil over a moderate heat. Ladle in 1/2 cup

(125ml) of the batter at a time, swirling to coat. Cook for 2 minutes, then flip gently and cook for 1 minute more. Repeat to make eight crepes.

3   Meanwhile, toss the broccolini in the olive oil, then cook on a hot ribbed grill for 4 minutes, until lightly blackened.

4   Spread the crepes with the hummus and sour cream, then top with the broccolini, spinach and chilli. Serve with soy bean and asparagus salad.

GREEN LINGUINE WITH RICOTTA, LEMON & BREADCRUMBS

Preparation time: 20 minutes • Cooking time: 20 minutes Serves: 4

Difficulty: ★★☆☆☆

1 bunch basil, leaves picked
1 bunch parsley, leaves picked
1 bunch marjoram, leaves picked
4 garlic cloves, peeled
1/2 cup (75g) toasted hazelnuts
1/2 cup (125ml) extra virgin olive oil
sea salt flakes and freshly ground
black pepper
1 1/2 cups (90g) fresh breadcrumbs
400g linguine
1 cup (250g) full-cream ricotta
finely grated zest of 4 lemons
basil leaves, to serve

1 Combine the herbs, garlic, hazelnuts and olive oil in a blender, then purée until smooth. Season with salt and pepper.

2 Put the breadcrumbs in a large non-stick frying pan over a moderate heat. Cook, tossing regularly, for a few minutes, until browned. Set aside.

3 Cook the pasta in a large saucepan of salted rapidly boiling water according to the packet instructions until al dente, then drain well.

4 Toss the pasta with the sauce, ricotta, lemon zest and half the toasted breadcrumbs.

5 Serve topped with the remaining breadcrumbs and basil.

DINNER

GRASS-FED LAMB LOIN CHOPS WITH WHOLE-WHEAT KIMCHI DUMPLINGS IN PEA & GARLIC HASH

Preparation time: 20 minutes • Cooking time: 20 minutes Serves: 4

Difficulty: ★★★☆☆

8 lamb loin chops
1 teaspoon celery salt
2 red onions, sliced
2 celery stalks, sliced
6 garlic cloves, sliced
1 bunch sage, sliced
1/4 cup (60ml) extra virgin olive oil
2 medium potatoes, peeled and grated
1 cup (250ml) beef stock

sea salt flakes and freshly ground
black pepper
1 1/2 cups (200g) frozen peas
1 bunch parsley, finely chopped
2 eggs
1 tablespoon kimchi, finely chopped
1 cup (150g) wholemeal flour

1   Season the chops with the celery salt, then
    set aside for 5 minutes. Sauté the onions,
    celery, garlic and sage in the olive oil over
    a moderate heat for 5 minutes, until softened,
    then add the potatoes and cook for 3
    minutes more. Pour in the stock, season with
    salt and pepper, then simmer until thickened.
    Mix in the peas and parsley.
2   Meanwhile, mix the eggs, kimchi and 1/2 cup
    (125ml) water in a bowl, whisking well. Add
    the flour and stir until thickened. Shape into
    12 small balls and cook in a saucepan of
    salted simmering water until the balls have
    floated for 3 minutes of cooking.
3   While the dumplings cook, fry the lamb chops
    on a hot ribbed griddle for 3 minutes on
    each side, until medium-rare.
4   Put the pea hash into bowls, then top with
    the chops and dumplings.

RAINBOW TROUT 'AL CARTOCCIO' WITH KIMCHI, BROCCOLINI, HEART OF PALM & CITRUS SALSA

Preparation time: 20 minutes • Cooking time: 20 minutes Serves: 4

Difficulty: ★★★☆☆

4 rainbow trout, butterflied [4]
sea salt flakes and freshly ground black pepper
1/4 cup (35g) kimchi, very finely chopped
1 tablespoon sriracha sauce
4 garlic cloves, minced
4cm piece of fresh ginger, grated
2 bunches broccolini, trimmed

---

[4] Ask your fishmonger to do this for you, or sandwich together pairs of trout fillets.

1 cup (150g) hearts of palm, finely sliced
2 kaffir lime leaves, very finely sliced
1/2 cup each segments of orange, lemon, lime and pink grapefruit
1 Lebanese cucumber, seeded and finely diced
1 red onion, very finely chopped
1/4 bunch mint, leaves chopped
2 tablespoons extra virgin olive oil

1 Season the trout generously with salt and pepper. Mix the kimchi, sriracha, garlic and ginger together, then stuff into each trout with the broccolini, hearts of palm and lime leaves. Wrap each fish separately in baking paper and a triple layer of foil, then arrange on a moderate heat barbecue grill and cook for 8 minutes on each side.

2 Meanwhile, mix the citrus, cucumber, onion and mint with the olive oil and season with salt and pepper.

3 Unwrap the trout parcels and serve with the salsa.

LINGUINE 'AGLIO E OLIO'

Preparation time: 10 minutes • Cooking time: 20 minutes Serves: 4

Difficulty: ★★☆☆☆

500g linguine
1/2 cup (125ml) extra virgin olive oil
1 1/2 cups (90g) fresh multigrain
breadcrumbs
10 garlic cloves, minced
1 1/2 teaspoons chilli flakes
finely grated zest of 2 lemons
2 rosemary sprigs, leaves finely
chopped
1 bunch parsley, very finely chopped
sea salt flakes and freshly ground
black pepper
finely grated pecorino cheese, to serve

1 Cook the pasta in a large saucepan of rapidly boiling salted water according to the packet instructions, until al dente. Drain well and toss with 2 tablespoons of the olive oil.

2   Meanwhile, fry the breadcrumbs in a large pan set over a moderate heat, until well-toasted and aromatic. Remove and set aside.

3   Pour the remaining oil into the pan and cook the garlic, chilli, lemon zest and rosemary for 5 minutes, until aromatic.

4   Mix in the pasta, breadcrumbs and parsley. Season with salt and pepper and serve sprinkled with pecorino.

PRAWN & ONION KEBABS WITH GRILLED CORN & BEAN SALAD

Preparation time: 15 minutes • Cooking time: 20 minutes Serves: 4

Difficulty: ★★☆☆☆

16 extra-large raw king prawns, peeled and deveined
1 red onion, cut into wedges
4 green shallots, cut into 4cm lengths
4 corn cobs
1/4 cup (60ml) extra virgin olive oil
2 cups green beans
4 ripe tomatoes, seeded and diced
400g can black-eyed beans, drained and rinsed
2 cups (80g) torn radicchio
sea salt flakes and freshly ground black pepper
2 tablespoons green goddess dressing
1 cup (30g) croutons

1   Thread the prawns, onion and shallots onto skewers and set aside.

2   Toss the corn in half the olive oil and cook on a hot barbecue grill for 10 minutes, turning often, until lightly blackened. Slice into rings.

3   Blanch the green beans in a pot of boiling water, then add to the corn with the tomatoes, black-eyed beans and radicchio. Season with salt and pepper, drizzle with the green goddess dressing and scatter with croutons.

4   Drizzle the skewers with the remaining oil and cook on a hot barbecue grill for 5 minutes, until firm.

5   Serve the skewers with the salad.

BAHARAT KOFTE WITH GOLDEN ROASTED BRUSSELS SPROUTS

Preparation time: 15 minutes • Cooking time: 45 minutes Serves: 4

Difficulty: ★★☆☆☆

600g beef mince
2 red onions, very finely diced
8 garlic cloves, minced
1/2 bunch dill, very finely chopped
1/2 cup breadcrumbs
1 1/2 tablespoons baharat spice mix [5]
1/2 teaspoon bicarbonate of soda
sea salt flakes and freshly ground black pepper
500g Brussels sprouts
2 green shallots, cut into 3cm pieces
1 bunch thyme, leaves picked
1/2 cup (125ml) extra virgin olive oil
1/2 cup (60g) walnuts, chopped

---

[5] Baharat is a Lebanese seven-spice mix available from good greengrocers and delicatessens.

juice of 1 lemon
yoghurt, chopped coriander and lemon
wedges, to serve

1   Preheat the oven to 180°C. Combine the mince, half the onion and garlic, all the dill, breadcrumbs, spice mix and bicarbonate of soda in a bowl. Season generously with salt and pepper. Knead until smooth, then thread onto 12 skewers.

2   Quarter the Brussels sprouts and toss with the shallots, thyme, remaining onion and garlic. Season with salt and pepper, drizzle with half the olive oil, then arrange on an oven tray. Roast for 45 minutes, until golden. Toss the walnuts and lemon juice through.

3   Meanwhile, drizzle the skewers with the remaining oil, then cook on a hot ribbed grill for 10 minutes, turning often, until firm to touch.

4   Serve the kofte on the Brussels sprouts, with yoghurt, coriander and lemon wedges.

SLOW-COOKED LAMB SHOULDER

Preparation time: 10 minutes • Cooking time: 3 hours Serves: 6

Difficulty: ★★★☆☆

**1.6kg lamb shoulder
sea salt flakes and freshly ground
black pepper
2 tablespoons extra virgin olive oil
6 celery stalks
2 whole garlic bulbs, halved
4 rosemary sprigs
2 cinnamon sticks
1 litre (4 cups) chicken stock
2 tablespoons plain flour
2 tablespoons unsalted butter, at
room temperature
greens and lemon wedges, to serve**

1   Preheat the oven to 220°C. Season the lamb generously with salt and pepper, then rub with the olive oil. Put the celery, garlic, rosemary and cinnamon in a roasting pan, then arrange the lamb on top.

2   Bake for 30 minutes, then pour in the stock and cover with foil. Turn the oven down to 150°C and bake for 21/2 hours. Remove from the oven, cover loosely with foil and leave to rest while making the gravy.

3   Strain the baking liquid into a saucepan and bring to a simmer. Mix the flour and butter to a paste, then whisk it into the pan 1 teaspoon at a time, until the sauce has thickened. (You may not need all the butter mixture, depending on how much liquid has evaporated during baking.)

4   Carve the lamb and serve with the gravy, greens and lemon wedges.

ROASTED MUSHROOM RISOTTO

Preparation time: 20 minutes • Cooking time: 45 minutes Serves: 4–6

Difficulty: ★★★☆☆

**1kg flat mushrooms
1/2 bunch thyme, leaves picked
2 teaspoons fennel seeds, cracked
10 garlic cloves, minced
3/4 cup (185ml) extra virgin olive oil
2 leeks, pale parts very finely diced
1/2 fennel bulb, very finely chopped
1 1/2 cups (330g) arborio rice
1 cup (250ml) white wine
3 cups (750ml) chicken stock, hot
3 tablespoons unsalted butter, at
room temperature
120g pecorino cheese, finely grated
sea salt flakes and freshly ground
black pepper
1 bunch dill, chopped**

1   Preheat the oven to 180°C. Arrange the mushrooms on a lined oven tray. Mix the

thyme, fennel seeds, half the garlic and 1/2 cup (125ml) of the olive oil in a bowl, then drizzle over the mushrooms. Bake for 40 minutes, until well softened. Chop roughly.

2   Meanwhile, sauté the leeks, fennel and remaining garlic in the remaining oil for 5 minutes over a moderate heat, until softened. Add the rice and cook for another 3 minutes. Pour in the wine and simmer for 3 minutes.

3   Add the stock one cup at a time, stirring very gently just once afterwards, allowing the stock to be absorbed before adding more.

4   When the liquid is almost all absorbed, add the butter and cheese, season with salt and pepper, then beat well until creamy. Fold in the mushrooms and dill.

CICERI E TRIA: PUGLIESE PASTA & CHICKPEAS

Preparation time: 15 minutes • Cooking time: 20 minutes Serves: 4

Difficulty: ★★☆☆☆

1 brown onion, very finely diced
2 celery stalks, very finely diced
8 garlic cloves, crushed
2 long red chillies, seeded and finely chopped
2 fresh bay leaves
1 teaspoon fennel seeds, cracked
1/2 cup (125ml) extra virgin olive oil
4 ripe tomatoes, seeded and diced
1 cup (250ml) white wine
sea salt flakes and freshly ground black pepper
2x400g cans chickpeas, drained
300g orecchiette
finely grated pecorino cheese and chopped parsley, to serve

1   Sauté the onion, celery, garlic, chillies, bay leaves and fennel seeds in the olive oil over a moderate heat for **8** minutes, until softened. Add the tomatoes and wine, season with salt and pepper, then simmer gently. Fold in the chickpeas.

2   Meanwhile, cook the pasta in a large saucepan of rapidly boiling salted water according to the packet instructions until al dente, then drain well.

3   Toss the pasta with the sauce, mixing in some pecorino, parsley and a generous amount of black pepper to serve.

VEGETARIAN MASSAMAN CURRY OF POTATOES, CELERY & TOFU

Preparation time: 20 minutes • Cooking time: 45 minutes Serves: 4–6

Difficulty: ★★★☆☆

6 French shallots, finely sliced
6 garlic cloves, finely sliced
6cm piece of fresh ginger, cut into fine batons
4 kaffir lime leaves, finely sliced
4 cinnamon sticks
I teaspoon cumin seeds
I teaspoon coriander seeds
12 cardamom pods, cracked
2 tablespoons sesame oil
1/2 cup (130g) red curry paste
1/4 cup (60ml) coconut aminos
1/4 cup (70g) peanut butter
I tablespoon ground turmeric
I litre (4 cups) vegetable stock

2x400ml cans coconut cream
6 medium potatoes, peeled and
chopped
4 celery stalks, chopped
400g firm tofu, diced
sea salt flakes and freshly ground
black pepper
coriander, lime wedges and toasted
coconut, to serve

1   Fry the shallots, garlic, ginger, lime leaves and spices in the sesame oil in a large saucepan over a moderate heat for 10 minutes, until softened. Stir in the curry paste, coconut aminos, peanut butter and turmeric, then fry for 2 minutes more.

2   Pour in the stock and coconut cream, then bring to a simmer. Add the potatoes, celery and tofu and simmer gently until the potatoes are tender. Season with salt and pepper.

3   Serve with coriander, lime wedges and toasted coconut.

ROASTED MACKEREL IN GREEN HERB CRUST

Preparation time: 15 minutes + 20 minutes
resting Cooking time: 20 minutes • Serves: 4

Difficulty: ★★★☆☆

4x180g mackerel cutlets
sea salt flakes and freshly ground
black pepper
1/2 cup (125ml) coconut vinegar
1/2 cup (125ml) extra virgin olive oil
1 bunch chives
1/2 bunch parsley
1/2 bunch dill
1/4 cup (35g) pistachios
4 garlic cloves, minced
1/2 cup (50g) finely grated parmesan
1/4 cup (15g) fresh multigrain
breadcrumbs
zest and juice of 2 lemons
baby salad leaves, to serve

1   Preheat the oven to 180°C. Season the fish
     generously with salt and pepper, douse with

the coconut vinegar, then set aside for 20 minutes. Drain off the excess liquid.

2 Pour 1 tablespoon of the olive oil into a large non-stick frying pan set over a high heat and sear the fish on both sides. Transfer to a roasting dish.

3 Combine the herbs, pistachios, garlic, parmesan, breadcrumbs, lemon zest and juice with the remaining oil in a food processor and purée until a paste forms. Spread onto the fish.

4 Bake for 10 minutes, until the fish is firm to touch. Serve with a baby leaf salad.

FLORENTINE-STYLE BARBECUED T-BONE WITH HERB BUTTER

Preparation time: 10 minutes + overnight marinating Cooking time: 20 minutes • Serves: 4

Difficulty: ★★☆☆☆

4 thick-cut T-bone steaks
1/4 cup (60ml) extra virgin olive oil
4 rosemary sprigs, leaves finely chopped
1 1/2 teaspoons fennel seeds, cracked
200g unsalted butter
1 tablespoon Worcestershire sauce
1/2 bunch thyme, finely chopped
1/2 bunch parsley, finely chopped
1/2 bunch chives, snipped
sea salt flakes and freshly ground white pepper
lemon wedges, to serve

1 Combine the steaks with the olive oil, rosemary and fennel seeds in a tray. Cover with plastic wrap, then refrigerate overnight.

2   Using a stand mixer, beat the butter, Worcestershire sauce and herbs on medium speed for 10 minutes, until smooth and light. Season with salt and pepper.

3   Season the steaks with salt and pepper, then cook on a hot barbecue grill for 12 minutes, turning several times, until medium-rare.

4   Rest the steaks for 3 minutes, then serve with the herb butter and lemon wedges.

BRAISED & CHARGRILLED OCTOPUS WITH GARDEN CRUDITÉS

Preparation time: 15 minutes + 2 hours resting
Cooking time: 45 minutes • Serves: 4

Difficulty: ★★★☆☆

1kg baby octopus, cleaned
2 brown onions, finely diced
6 garlic cloves, minced
4 fresh bay leaves
4 juniper berries
1/2 cup (125ml) extra virgin olive oil
2 cups (500ml) dry white wine
1 litre (4 cups) chicken stock
sea salt flakes and freshly ground
black pepper
cucumber, carrots and fennel, cut into
fine batons
tzatziki, grilled flatbread and mint
leaves, to serve

1   Pat the octopus dry with paper towel.
2   Sauté the onions, garlic, bay leaves and juniper berries in 2 tablespoons of the olive oil in a large saucepan over a moderate heat for 5 minutes, until softened. Add the wine and simmer for 5 minutes. Pour in the stock and bring to a simmer.
3   Add the octopus, then simmer very gently for 20 minutes. Turn the heat off and allow to cool. Drain the octopus, then refrigerate for 2 hours, until firm.
4   Toss the octopus in the remaining oil and season with salt and pepper. Cook over a hot barbecue grill for 5 minutes, until lightly blackened.
5   Serve with the vegetable batons, tzatziki, flatbread and mint.

GRILLED CHICKEN & TOMATO WHITE CORN TOSTADAS

Preparation time: 15 minutes • Cooking time: 1 hour Serves: 4

Difficulty: ★★☆☆☆

**4 ripe tomatoes, quartered
sea salt flakes and freshly ground
black pepper
1 bunch thyme, finely chopped
2 teaspoons red wine vinegar
4 chicken breast fillets
1/2 cup (125ml) extra virgin olive oil
finely grated zest and juice of 2 limes
1 teaspoon ground cumin
1/2 teaspoon ground coriander
1/2 teaspoon ground chilli
1/2 teaspoon ground allspice
12 small white corn tacos
vegetable oil, for deep-frying
2 cups (150g) shredded green cabbage
2 avocados, flesh crushed**

hot sauce, coriander and sour cream, to serve

1 Preheat the oven to 140°C. Season the tomatoes with salt and pepper, then sprinkle with the thyme and vinegar. Arrange on a rack over an oven tray and place in a lidded BBQ set to moderate for 1 hour, until half dried.

2 Meanwhile, toss the chicken in half the olive oil and season with salt and pepper. Cook over a barbecue grill for 15 minutes, until just firm. Slice finely, then toss with the lime zest and juice, spices and remaining oil.

3 Drizzle the tacos with vegetable oil, then cook on the BBQ flat plate until crisp, then drain on paper towel.

4 Top the tacos with the cabbage, avocado, chicken, tomatoes, hot sauce, coriander and sour cream.

KOREAN-STYLE BRAISED BEEF SHORT RIBS

Preparation time: 20 minutes • Cooking time: 4 hours Serves: 4

Difficulty: ★★★★☆

1.5kg beef short ribs, cut into four pieces by your butcher
sea salt flakes and freshly ground black pepper
2 tablespoons extra virgin olive oil
6 celery stalks, trimmed
2 cups (500ml) beef stock
1/4 cup (60ml) gochujang sauce
1/4 cup (60ml) soy sauce
1/4 cup (60ml) sesame oil
1/4 cup (45g) dark brown sugar
1 brown onion, grated
6 garlic cloves, minced
6cm piece of fresh ginger, grated
sliced green onions, coriander, sesame seeds and rice, to serve

1 Preheat the oven to 150°C.
2 Season the beef ribs with salt and pepper, then toss with the olive oil. Sear in a heavy-based pan over a high heat until browned. Set the ribs on a bed of celery stalks in a roasting pan and pour in the stock.
3 Mix together the gochujang and soy sauces, sesame oil, sugar, onion, garlic and ginger, then spread over the beef. Cover with baking paper and foil, then bake for 3 hours, until the beef is tender.
4 Remove the foil and paper, increase the oven temperature to 200°C, then bake for a further 30 minutes, until glazed.
5 Serve with green onions, coriander, sesame seeds and rice.

DESSERTS & SNACKS

SUGAR-FREE RYE & BERRY SHORTCAKES WITH YOGHURT

Preparation time: 15 minutes • Cooking time: 20 minutes Serves: 4

Difficulty: ★★☆☆☆

1 cup (150g) self-raising flour
1 cup (120g) rye flour
1 1/2 teaspoons baking powder
1/2 teaspoon fine salt
2 tablespoons monkfruit powder
125g cold unsalted butter, grated
2 cups (500g) Greek style yoghurt
finely grated zest of 2 oranges
3cm piece of fresh ginger, finely grated
300ml cream, whipped to soft peaks
2 cups (400g) mixed fresh berries

1   Preheat the oven to 180°C. Combine the flours, baking powder, salt and monkfruit powder in a food processor and pulse to combine. Add the butter and pulse again. Add 1 1/3 cups (325g) of the yoghurt, the orange zest and ginger, then pulse until a rough dough forms.

2   Divide the dough into four pieces and gently form into balls. Arrange on a lined oven tray and bake for 18–20 minutes, until golden. Cool on a wire rack.

3   Split the shortcakes, then fill with the whipped cream and berries. Spread the remaining yoghurt on plates, then put the shortcakes on top.

SIMPLE VANILLA-LEMON-RICOTTA CHEESECAKE WITH CHERRY COMPOTE

Preparation time: 15 minutes • Cooking time: 40 minutes Serves: 10

Difficulty: ★★★☆☆

250g packet butternut snap biscuits
75g unsalted butter, melted
8 eggs
500g ricotta cheese
finely grated zest of 2 lemons
2 teaspoons vanilla bean paste
3/4 cup (185ml) light honey
2 cups (300g) fresh or frozen pitted cherries
whipped cream, to serve

1 Preheat the oven to 160°C. Crush the biscuits into a coarse powder, then mix with the butter and 2 egg whites. Press into the

bottom of a lined 20cm cake tin and bake for 8 minutes.

2   Combine the ricotta, lemon zest, vanilla and 1/2 cup (125ml) of the honey in a food processor and purée until smooth. Add the remaining eggs and egg yolks and purée thoroughly. Pour over the biscuit base, then bake for 30–40 minutes, until just firm.

3   Meanwhile, mix the cherries and remaining honey in a small saucepan over a very low heat. Cook gently for 10 minutes, until the cherries are almost tender. Set aside to cool.

4   Serve the cherry compote with the cheesecake and whipped cream.

MIXED MELON SALAD WITH LIME & MARJORAM

Preparation time: 15 minutes • Cooking time: 5 minutes Serves: 4

Difficulty: ★★☆☆☆

3 cups watermelon, in balls
2 cups rockmelon, in balls
1 cup honeydew melon, in balls
1 cup Piel de Sapo melon, in balls
3/4 cup coconut shavings
10 limes
1/2 cup (125ml) light honey
2 fresh bay leaves
2 fennel seeds
2 bunches marjoram, leaves picked

1   Combine the melons and coconut in a bowl and toss gently.
2   Cut 4 limes into segments and mix with the melons, then juice the remaining limes.
3   Mix the lime juice, honey, bay leaves and fennel seeds in a small saucepan and boil for

5 minutes, until thickened. Strain through a fine sieve, then allow to cool.

4 Mix the syrup and marjoram through the melons.

EASY OLIVE OIL CHOCOLATE-CHUNK COOKIES

Preparation time: 10 minutes • Cooking time: 20 minutes Makes: about 48

Difficulty: ★★☆☆☆

3/4 cup (185ml) extra virgin olive oil
1 cup (200g) stevia powder
1/2 cup (125ml) molasses
2 eggs
2 egg yolks
1 1/2 teaspoons vanilla bean paste
1 teaspoon almond essence
1 3/4 cups (260g) plain flour
1 cup (130g) buckwheat flour
1 1/2 teaspoons ground cinnamon
1/2 teaspoon ground nutmeg
1 teaspoon baking powder
3/4 teaspoon bicarbonate of soda
1/2 cup (125ml) buttermilk
300g sugar-free dark chocolate (70% cocoa), chopped into chunks
2 teaspoons sea salt flakes

1 Preheat the oven to 170°C. Combine the olive oil, stevia, molasses, eggs, yolks, vanilla and almond essence in a bowl and whisk until the sugar has dissolved.

2 Sift the flours, spices, baking powder and bicarbonate of soda together, then gently fold into the egg mixture. Mix in the buttermilk and chocolate.

3 Place tablespoon amounts on lined oven trays and sprinkle with the salt.

4 Bake for 18–20 minutes, until just firm halfway to the centre. Cool on a wire rack.

DATE, MACADAMIA & CINNAMON ROLLS

Preparation time: 30 minutes + 2 hours proving
Cooking time: 30 minutes • Makes: 12

Difficulty: ★★★★☆

31/3 cups (500g) bakers' flour [6]
2 teaspoons bread improver
2 teaspoons ground turmeric
10g (1 1/2 sachets) instant dried yeast
3/4 cup (150g) monkfruit powder
4 egg yolks
100g unsalted butter, at room
temperature
1 1/2 teaspoons fine salt
300g dried dates
1 teaspoon bicarbonate of soda
100g (2/3 cup) macadamias, toasted
and finely chopped
2 teaspoons ground cinnamon
1/4 cup (60ml) maple syrup

---

[6] Bakers' flour is flour with a higher protein count,
making it perfect for making breads, pizzas and sweet
rolls.

1 Combine the flour, bread improver, turmeric, yeast and 1/4 cup (50g) of the monkfruit powder in the bowl of a stand mixer and mix well. With the motor running on low speed, add 450ml tepid water, then add the egg yolks and the butter one teaspoon at a time. Mix in the salt, then knead until smooth.

2 Cover the dough with plastic wrap and set aside for 1 hour, until doubled in size. Meanwhile, put the dates and bicarbonate of soda in a bowl and cover with boiling water. Stand for 5 minutes, then drain well and crush the dates.

3 Roll out the dough to make a 30cm x 25cm rectangle. Spread with the date paste, leaving a 5cm margin at the far edge. Top with the macadamias, cinnamon and remaining monkfruit powder, then roll up, finishing with the clean edge.

4 Slice into 12 discs, then arrange on a lined oven tray, tucking the clean edge underneath. Cover with plastic wrap and set aside for 1 hour, until nearly doubled in size.

5 Preheat the oven to 200°C. Bake the rolls for 10 minutes, then turn the oven down to 170°C and bake for 15 minutes more.

6 Brush the rolls with maple syrup as soon as they come out of the oven.

HOMEMADE CHEESE STICKS

Preparation time: 10 minutes • Cooking time: 25 minutes Makes: 12

Difficulty: ★★☆☆☆

300g best-quality puff pastry (or 4 sheets)
2 eggs, beaten
200g mozzarella, grated
100g pecorino, finely grated
100g Stilton, crumbled
1 1/2 teaspoons mixed dried herbs
sea salt flakes and freshly ground black pepper

1   Preheat the oven to 200°C. Roll out the pastry to 3mm thick, if not using sheets. Brush both sides with the eggs. Mix the cheeses and press into the pastry on both sides. Scatter with dried herbs and season with salt and pepper.
2   Slice into 12 strips, 3cm wide, then twist each and arrange on lined biscuit trays.

3   Bake for 22–25 minutes, until deep golden and crisp. Cool on a wire rack.

WHIPPED VANILLA CUSTARD WITH APRICOTS & CRISP PARMESAN-WALNUT WAFERS

Preparation time: 15 minutes • Cooking time: 30 minutes Serves: 4

Difficulty: ★★★☆☆

2 cups (500ml) milk
4 eggs
1/2 cup (100g) stevia powder
40g (1/3 cup) cornflour
1 teaspoon vanilla bean paste
1 teaspoon almond essence
400ml whipping cream
1 cup poached or tinned apricots
(approx. 16 apricot halves)
1 tablespoon unsalted butter, melted
1/4 cup (35g) plain flour
1/4 cup (25g) grated parmesan
2 tablespoons finely chopped walnuts

1 Bring the milk to a simmer in a small saucepan over a moderate heat.

2 Meanwhile, crack 2 eggs into a bowl. Add the yolks from the remaining 2 eggs, reserving the whites. Add the stevia, cornflour, vanilla and almond essence and whisk until smooth.

3 Mix the hot milk through the egg mixture. Pour into a clean saucepan and simmer over a moderate heat until thickened. Cover with plastic wrap and set aside to cool completely.

4 Whip the cream to stiff peaks, then fold it through the custard. Put the apricots in four glasses and top with the custard.

5 Meanwhile, preheat the oven to 180°C. Beat the egg whites, butter, flour and parmesan in a bowl until smooth. Spread thinly on lined biscuit trays, then scatter with walnuts. Bake for 8 minutes, until browned.

6 Serve the wafers with the custard.

MOCHA CAKE WITH CAROB SYRUP & GRAPE SALAD

Preparation time: 10 minutes • Cooking time: 55 minutes Serves: 10

Difficulty: ★★★☆☆

125g unsalted butter
125g coconut oil
250g sugar-free dark chocolate, chopped
2 teaspoons vanilla extract
1/2 teaspoon fine salt
1 tablespoon instant coffee powder
1 1/4 cups (310ml) monkfruit syrup
6 eggs, 4 separated
1 cup (100g) cocoa powder
2 cups (360g) grapes, quartered
300g fior di latte cheese, torn
1 cup (190g) pineapple, finely diced
1/4 cup (40g) toasted pine nuts, chopped

carob syrup, to serve [7]

1 Preheat the oven to 180°C. Put in a medium saucepan, over a moderate heat, cook the butter until browned. Stir in the coconut oil and set aside to cool slightly. Add the chocolate, vanilla, salt, coffee powder and monkfruit syrup, stirring until smooth.

2 Whisk in 2 eggs and 4 egg yolks, then sift in the cocoa powder. Whisk the egg whites to soft peaks and fold in. Spoon into a lined 22cm cake tin and bake for 45–50 minutes, until just firm to touch. Cool in the tin.

3 Mix the grapes, cheese, pineapple and pine nuts.

4 Serve slices of cake with the grape salad and carob syrup.

---

[7] Carob pods are about 50% sugar by weight, cooked down to a traditional syrup in Malta and Cyprus. Mostly fructose and glucose, it is offset by naturally occurring fibre. Carob syrup is available at continental delis or online.

DANISH BUTTER BISCUITS

Preparation time: 15 minutes + freezing Cooking
time: 15 minutes • Makes: about 48

Difficulty: ★★★☆☆

125g unsalted butter, melted
1/2 cup (100g) stevia powder
1 teaspoon vanilla bean paste
1 egg
1 egg yolk
1 cup (100g) almond meal
2 tablespoons plain flour
1/2 teaspoon xanthan gum [8]
48 blanched almonds

1   Combine the butter, stevia and vanilla in a
bowl and whisk thoroughly, then beat in the
egg and egg yolk. Mix the almond meal, flour
and xanthan gum in a bowl, then fold into
the butter mixture.

---

[8] Xanthan gum is a type of sugar that's commonly used
as a food additive to thicken, emulsify and/or stabilise,
preventing ingredients from separating.

2   Load into a piping bag fitted with a 1cm star nozzle, then pipe as rosettes onto lined oven trays. Top each with an almond. Freeze, until firm.

3   Preheat the oven to 180°C. Bake the biscuits for 9–12 minutes, until golden. Cool on a wire rack.

CAFFÈ CORRETTO PANNA COTTA WITH TWICE-COOKED BERRIES

Preparation time: 10 minutes + 3 hours chilling
Cooking time: 15 minutes • Serves: 4

Difficulty: ★★★★☆

20g gelatine powder
350ml milk
1/4 cup (50g) stevia powder
1 1/2 tablespoons instant coffee powder
300ml thickened cream
50ml Frangelico
1 cup (250ml) strong espresso coffee
1 cinnamon stick
2 star anise
1 cup (250ml) monkfruit syrup
2 cups (400g) mixed fresh or frozen berries

1   Mix the gelatine with 1/4 cup (60ml) cold water and set aside for 5 minutes. Meanwhile, pour the milk into a medium saucepan, stir in the stevia and coffee powder and bring to a simmer over a low heat. Stir in the gelatine, then set aside to cool.

2   Strain the coffee mixture through a fine sieve into the cream and Frangelico. Stir gently, pour into four moulds and refrigerate for 3 hours.

3   Pour the espresso into a small saucepan. Add the spices and half the monkfruit syrup and simmer for 5 minutes. Strain through a fine sieve and allow to cool.

4   Put 1/2 cup berries in a small saucepan with the remaining monkfruit syrup and 1/4 cup (60ml) water. Boil rapidly for 3 minutes. While hot, strain through a fine sieve and mix with the remaining berries. Cover with plastic wrap and allow to steep gently.

5   Dip the moulds in hot water, then invert onto cold plates and unmould. Drizzle with the syrup and serve with the berries.

BROWN BUTTER & RASPBERRY CAKE

Preparation time: 10 minutes • Cooking time: 45 minutes Serves: 10

Difficulty: ★★★☆☆

450g unsalted butter, at room temperature
200ml maple syrup
5 eggs
2 egg yolks
1 cup (250ml) monkfruit syrup
1 tablespoon vanilla bean paste
2 1/4 cups (335g) plain flour
3 teaspoons baking powder
1 cup (250ml) buttermilk
2 punnets raspberries
raspberries and toasted hazelnuts, to decorate

1 Preheat the oven to 180°C. Line a lined medium loaf pan with baking paper.
2 Melt 350g of the butter in a medium saucepan over a moderate heat until it turns foamy and smells of hazelnuts. Put the

bottom of the pan in a bowl of cold water to stop the cooking. Allow to cool.

3   Combine the remaining butter in a bowl with the maple syrup, eggs, egg yolks, 150ml of the monkfruit syrup and half the vanilla and whisk until very smooth. Sift the flour and baking powder together, then fold in with 3/4 cup (185ml) of the buttermilk, then mix gently. Fold in the raspberries, then spoon into the lined loaf pan.

4   Bake for 40 minutes, until a skewer can be inserted and removed cleanly. Cool on a wire rack.

5   Put the remaining butter, monkfruit syrup, vanilla and buttermilk in the bowl of a stand mixer. Using the paddle attachment, beat on medium speed until very light.

6   Spread the frosting on the cake, then decorate with raspberries and hazelnuts.

EASY LEMON TEA CAKE

Preparation time: 15 minutes • Cooking time: 45 minutes Serves: 10

Difficulty: ★★☆☆☆

> **175g unsalted butter**
> **150ml monkfruit syrup**
> **finely grated zest and juice of 4 lemons**
> **2 teaspoons ground turmeric**
> **2 eggs**
> **2 egg yolks**
> **1/2 cup (125ml) buttermilk**
> **225g (1 1/2 cups) self-raising flour**
> **1 teaspoon baking powder**
> **whipped cream and strawberry salad, to serve**

1   Preheat the oven to 180°C. Line a medium loaf pan with baking paper.
2   Put the butter in the bowl of a stand mixer and beat with the paddle attachment on medium speed for 3 minutes, until light. Add 100ml of the monkfruit syrup, the lemon zest and turmeric, then beat for another 3 minutes.

3   With the motor running, add the eggs, egg yolks, buttermilk and half the lemon juice. Once smooth, reduce the speed to low. Sift the flour and baking powder in, mixing until smooth.

4   Spoon into a lined medium loaf pan and bake for 40–45 minutes, until a skewer can be inserted and removed cleanly.

5   Put the remaining lemon juice and monkfruit syrup in a small saucepan over a moderate heat. Simmer for 3 minutes, then drizzle over the cake.

6   Serve with whipped cream and strawberry salad.

SUGAR-FREE CROSTOLI

Preparation time: 10 minutes + 1 hour chilling
Cooking time: 5 minutes • Makes: about 24

Difficulty: ★★☆☆☆

2 cups (300g) plain flour
1/2 cup (75g) self-raising flour
1/2 cup (55g) coconut flour
2 tablespoons stevia powder
finely grated zest and juice of 1 lemon
3 eggs
1/4 cup (60ml) dark rum
2 teaspoons vanilla bean paste
2 tablespoons extra virgin olive oil
vegetable oil, for deep-frying
stevia powder, for dusting

1 Combine the flours in a bowl and mix well. Add the stevia and lemon zest and stir thoroughly.
2 Whisk the eggs, lemon juice, rum, vanilla and olive oil in a second bowl, then add to the flour mix and stir until smooth. Refrigerate for 1 hour.
3 Roll out the dough to 3mm thick. Use a fluted rotary cutter or sharp knife to cut

rectangles measuring about 10cm x 3cm. Make a 6cm incision down the centre of each rectangle. Working with one piece at a time, loop one end through the hole and pull tight to make a twist.

4   Fry the strips in hot (180°C) vegetable oil for 2 minutes, until crisp and golden. Drain on paper towel.

5   Serve dusted with a little more stevia.

PEACH & ALMOND TART

Preparation time: 20 minutes + chilling Cooking time: 1 hour • Serves: 8–10

Difficulty: ★★★☆☆

300g shortcrust pastry
150g unsalted butter
2 cups (200g) almond meal
1 teaspoon ground cinnamon
4 eggs
4 egg yolks
100ml monkfruit syrup
finely grated zest of 2 oranges
1 teaspoon vanilla bean paste
1 teaspoon almond essence
1/4 cup (35g) gluten-free plain flour
8 poached peaches, tinned or bottled
1/2 cup (80g) blanched almonds
1/2 cup (165g) sugar-free peach jam
Light thickened cream and fresh raspberries, to serve

1 Roll out the pastry to a 30cm disc, then use it to line a 22cm tart tin. Chill for 20 minutes.

2 Preheat the oven to 180°C. Line the pastry base with foil and baking weights. Bake for 25 minutes, until golden and crisp. Remove the foil and weights.

3 Combine the butter, almond meal and cinnamon in the bowl of a stand mixer and beat with the paddle attachment on medium speed until smooth. Add the eggs, egg yolks, monkfruit syrup, orange zest, vanilla, almond essence and flour, then beat again.

4 Spoon into the pastry shell and smooth down evenly. Arrange the peaches and almonds on top. Bake for 30 minutes, until the filling is set. Allow to cool.

5 Boil the jam then brush over the top of the tart.

6 Serve with thickened cream and raspberries.

Dr Clare Bailey's

BONUS DAY OF RECIPES

Dr Clare Bailey's Nutrition Tip #12

Start your meal with a salad dressed with olive oil and live cider vinegar. This slows any sugar spikes with your main meal, helping to maintain healthy blood sugars as well as supporting a healthy gut microbiome.

SCRAMBLED EGGS ON SOURDOUGH TOAST WITH SMOKED SALMON & HOMEMADE SAUERKRAUT

This is our favourite family breakfast! It's easy to make, full of flavour and high in protein and omega-3, as well as providing plenty of fibre to keep your gut microbiome happy, thanks to the fermented sourdough and sauerkraut.

Preparation time: 5 minutes • Cooking time: 2 minutes Serves: 1

Difficulty: ★☆☆☆☆

1 thin slice of whole grain or seeded sourdough bread
1 knob of butter (or a dash of olive oil)
2 medium eggs
Small pinch of chilli flakes (optional)
80g sliced smoked salmon

40g of sauerkraut (ideally a red/purple version for colour)
Ground black pepper (to taste)

1 Toast the bread and spread with butter or non-dairy equivalent and place on the plate.
2 Whisk the eggs lightly with a fork in a cup or bowl.
3 Add the butter to a small non-stick pan over a gentle heat until it melts. Add the eggs and using a wooden spoon or spatula, stir slowly and steadily for 1–2 minutes to produce a creamy, slightly runny consistency. Remove from heat before it gets too firm.
4 Heap the scrambled eggs straight onto the toast and scatter with ground black pepper and a small pinch of chilli flakes, if using.
5 Place the salmon and the sauerkraut alongside and serve.

EASY MISO SOUP WITH PRAWNS & NOODLES (ADAPTED FROM THE FAST 800 EASY)

This makes a tasty yet quick and easy soup which is high in protein and surprisingly filling. The prawns are an excellent source of much-needed omega-3, the pak choi provides soluble fibre to feed the microbiome and the fermented miso paste adds extra nutrients and flavour.

Preparation time: 10 minutes • Cooking time: 10 minutes Serves: 2

Difficulty: ★☆☆☆☆

2 tablespoons miso paste (about 30g)
2 medium closed cup mushrooms, sliced (around 2–3mm thick)
2 small pak choi or 1 large, sliced into eighths lengthwise
30g of brown noodles or buckwheat soba noodles

150g large cooked peeled prawns (defrosted if frozen)
1 spring onion, finely chopped
1/2 tablespoon Thai fish sauce (optional)
pinch of dried chilli flakes to taste (optional)
Handful of coriander leaves

1 Pour 500ml hot water into a pan and bring to the boil, then add the miso paste, mushrooms and pak choi and bring to a simmer for 4–5 minutes.
2 Cook the noodles according to the instructions, run under cold water and set aside.
3 Add the prawns, spring onion, chilli flakes, fish sauce if using to the pan and cook for another couple of minutes until the prawns are heated through.
4 Remove from the heat, share between 2 deep bowls, season with ground black pepper and scatter with coriander leaves, and serve.

TIP

You can add spinach or cooked sliced greens instead of pak choi, and swap prawns for tofu if you like.

EASY MOROCCAN CHICKEN TAGINE

Tagine is a sweet and mildly spiced North African stew, cooked in an earthenware pot with a lid. All of the ingredients are traditionally thrown in the pot, right from the start, keeping only the coriander leaves for garnish at the end. Marinating and frying the chicken enhances the flavour a little, but I often simply throw it all in at once, give it a stir, cover with a well-fitting lid and put it straight in the oven for about an hour. This recipe looks like it involves a lot of ingredients, but it's really easy to prepare.

Preparation time: 10 minutes + marinating time
Cooking time: 1 hour and 20 minutes • Serves: 4–6

Difficulty: ★☆☆☆☆

6 skinless, boneless chicken thighs, diced into about 2–3cm chunks
2 teaspoons cumin seeds
2 teaspoons coriander
1 teaspoon turmeric
1 teaspoon cinnamon

1–1&1/2 teaspoons chilli flakes, to taste
4 tablespoons olive oil
2 large onions, finely diced
3cm fresh ginger, diced (or 1 teaspoon ground ginger)
3 garlic cloves, crushed and diced
2 red peppers, seeded and sliced
1 400g tin chopped tomatoes
1 chicken stock cube
1 400g tin chickpeas, drained
80g dried apricots, sliced
1 small lemon, washed, cut into quarters
60g pitted green olives
Generous handful of fresh coriander, stalks chopped

1 Marinate the chicken in a bowl, rubbing in the spices, and 1/2 teaspoon black pepper in a bowl and leave for 30–45 minutes at room temperature, or for 2–3 hours or overnight in the fridge.
2 Heat oven to 150°C.
3 Add the olive oil and spiced chicken to a large casserole with a well-fitting lid and fry the chicken for a few minutes over medium–high heat to lightly brown, stirring frequently.

4   Reduce the heat, add the onions and sweat for 3–4 minutes. Add the ginger and garlic, then cook for about a minute more.

5   Add the remaining ingredients, including the coriander stalks, but not the coriander leaves. Season with salt and generously with ground black pepper. Top up with 200–250ml water, cover and place in the oven for about 40 minutes, checking occasionally to see if extra water is needed to loosen.

6   Remove the lemon, stir in half the remaining coriander leaves and garnish with the rest.

7   Serve with quinoa or bulgur wheat if you like, along with freshly cooked greens and drizzle with full-fat live Greek yoghurt.

TIP

You don't need to have all of the spices – for ease you can replace the spices with 1 tablespoon ras el hanout (a Moroccan spice combination) or a 1–2 tablespoons of a good-quality harissa paste.

CHEESY PARMESAN BISCUITS WITH ROSEMARY

Ideal for a savoury snack, to provide the base of a light lunch, or even to grab as a breakfast or lunch on the run. High in protein, natural fat and fibre, these biscuits will also keep you full for longer. A treat that doesn't spike blood sugars!

Preparation time: 10 minutes • Cooking time: 12 minutes Serves: 20 biscuits

Difficulty: ★☆☆☆☆

100g parmesan, grated
100g cheddar
100g ground almonds
50g mixed seeds
1 sprig rosemary, finely chopped
(about 1 level dessert spoon)
1 egg white, lightly whisked

1   Preheat the oven to 170°C and line a large baking tray with baking paper.

2   Mix all the dry ingredients and the rosemary in a medium–large bowl. Then add the egg white and, using a wooden spoon, vigorously mix it to form a slightly crumbly dough. If it's too crumbly, add 1/2 tablespoon water and mix again so it holds together.

3   Scoop the mixture and press it firmly into a dessert spoon. With a dessert spoon in one hand, use your other hand to scoop the mixture and press it firmly into the spoon until it is almost level, then scoop it out and place it on the baking paper. Next, press them into shape and use a fork to press them to a thickness of no more than 1cm.

4   Place the tray in the middle of the oven. Check them within 10 minutes and every few minutes after. Remove from the oven when they are light golden brown around the edges. They usually take about 12 minutes. When ready, remove to a rack and allow to cool and firm up.

TIPS

You can use other robust herbs such as thyme or sage.

These would also work well baked in a tray as cheesy snack bars, though you would need to increase cooking time.

These biscuits can be kept in a container in the fridge for up to a week or can be frozen.

About the author

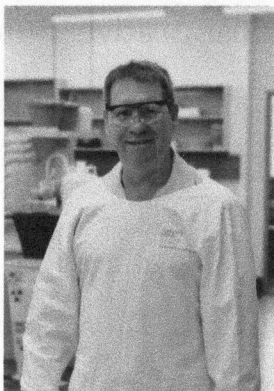

Professor Phil Hansbro is an internationally recognised research leader in the study of respiratory diseases, such as asthma, chronic obstructive airway disease (COPD, aka emphysema), idiopathic pulmonary fibrosis (IPF), and infections and is developing interests in lung cancer. His work is substantially contributing to understanding the pathogenesis and developing new therapies for these diseases.

His work has made internationally important contributions and led to the identification of novel avenues for therapy that are under further study. This is achieved through the development of novel mouse models that recapitulate the hallmark features of human disease, including infections, asthma, COPD, IPF and now lung cancer. He employs these models in integrated approaches (infection, immunity and physiology with particular expertise in lung function analysis) to understand human diseases, and develop new treatment strategies. Research outcomes have a translational goal and his studies are conducted in parallel with collaborative human studies with clinical researchers.

Contributors

Chapter 1: Inflammation overload – what it looks like, and why it matters
–Prof Phil Hansbro

Chapter 2: How does chronic inflammation cause disease?
–Prof Phil Hansbro, Dr Annalicia Vaughan

Chapter 3: Ageing and inflammation: inflammageing
–Prof David G. Le Couteur

Chapter 4: Welcome to the microbiome
–Dr SJ Shen, Prof Phil Hansbro

Chapter 5: How our gut microbiome influences inflammation
–A/Prof Laurence Macia, Prof Phil Hansbro

Chapter 6: How diet shapes our microbiome
–Dr Kurtis Budden, A/Prof Andy Holmes, Zhen Bao, Alison Luk, Prof Phil Hansbro

Chapter 7: The rise of the modern Western diet

–Prof Lisa Wood, Dr Annalicia Vaughan, Prof Phil Hansbro

Chapter 8: Minimising inflammation: lifestyle and microbiome approaches
–Prof Phil Hansbro

Chapter 9: What to eat – and why
–A/Prof Laurence Macia, Jordan Stanford, Prof Phil Hansbro

Chapter 10: Meal planner
–Fast Ed Halmagyi
Breakfast
Lunch
Dinner
Dessert & snacks

Nutrition Tips and Bonus Recipes
–Dr Clare Bailey

Endnotes

[1]   Jacka et al., 'A randomised controlled trial of dietary improvement for adults with major depression (the "SMILES" trial)'

[2]   Su et al., 'Remodeling of the gut microbiome during Ramadan-associated intermittent fasting'

[3]   Nunes, Pereira and Morais-Almeida, 'Asthma costs and social impact'

[4]   WHO, 'Chronic obstructive pulmonary disease (COPD)'

[5]   ERS, 'The economic burden of lung disease'

[6]   Allan and Arroll, 'Prevention and treatment of the common cold: making sense of the evidence'

[7]   Dadonaite and Roser, 'Pneumonia'

[8]   Su et al., 'Tracking total spending on tuberculosis by source and function in 135 low-income and middle-income countries, 2000–17: A financial modelling study'

[9]   AAAAI, 'Atopic march defined

[10]   Puac, '25 noteworthy allergy statistics & facts to know in 2022'

[11]   Puac, '25 noteworthy allergy statistics & facts to know in 2022'

[12]   Bilaver, 'Economic burden of food allergy: A systematic review'

[13]   Jean, 'Allergic rhinitis'

[14]   Mayo Clinic, 'Inflammatory bowel disease (IBD)'

[15]   Alatab et al., 'The global, regional, and national burden of inflammatory bowel disease in 195 countries and territories, 1990–2017: A systematic analysis for the Global Burden of Disease Study 2017'

[16]   Lichtenstein et al., 'Lifetime economic burden of Crohn's disease and ulcerative colitis by age at diagnosis'

[17]   Hoffman, 'Autoimmune disorders?'

[18]   AARDA and NCAPG, 'The cost burden of autoimmune disease: The latest front in the war on healthcare spending'

[19]   Feigin et al., 'Global, regional, and national burden of neurological disorders, 1990–2016: A systematic analysis for the Global Burden of Disease Study 2016'

[20]   Mindgardens, 'Review of the burden of disease for neurological, mental health and substance use disorders in Australia'

[21]   CDC, 'Stroke signs and symptoms'

[22]   Hur et al., 'The innate immunity protein IFITM3 modulates γ-secretase in Alzheimer's disease'

[23]   Caggiu et al., 'Inflammation, infectious triggers, and Parkinson's disease'

[24]   Valadãoa et al., 'Inflammation in Huntington's disease: A few new twists on an old tale'

[25]   Dinet et al., 'Brain–immune interactions and neuroinflammation after traumatic brain injury'

[26]   Better Health Channel, 'Pelvic inflammatory disease (PID)'

[27]   Sun et al., 'Global, regional, and national prevalence and disability-adjusted life-years for infertility in 195 countries and territories, 1990–2017: Results from a Global Burden of Disease Study, 2017'

[28]   Njagi et al., 'Economic costs of infertility care for patients in low-income and middle-income countries: A systematic review protocol'

[29]   Saad-Naguib et al., 'Cost-effective analysis of infertility treatment in women with anovulatory polycystic ovarian syndrome'

[30]   Davita Kidney Care, 'Anemia and chronic kidney disease'

[31]   National Kidney Foundation, 'Global facts: About kidney disease'

[32]   Healthgrades, 'Liver failure'

[33]   Asrani et al., 'Burden of liver diseases in the world'; Sepanlou et al., 'The

global, regional, and national burden of cirrhosis by cause in 195 countries and territories, 1990–2017: A systematic analysis for the Global Burden of Disease Study 2017'

[34]   Hirode et al., 'Trends in the burden of chronic liver disease among hospitalized US adults'

[35]   CTCA, 'Inflammation linked to cancer, but lifestyle changes may help'

[36]   CTCA, 'Inflammation linked to cancer, but lifestyle changes may help'

[37]   CTCA, 'Inflammation linked to cancer, but lifestyle changes may help'

[38]   National Cancer Institute, 'Symptoms of cancer'

[39]   WHO, 'Cancer'

[40]   Stewart and Wild (eds), 'World cancer report 2014'

[41]   Stewart and Wild (eds), 'World cancer report 2014'

[42]   Aristizábal and González, 'Innate immune system'

[43]   López-Otín et al., 'The hallmarks of aging'

[44]   Scudellari, 'To stay young, kill zombie cells'

[45]   Ferrucci and Fabbri, 'Inflammageing: Chronic inflammation in ageing, cardiovascular disease, and frailty'

[46]   Armanios et al., 'Translational strategies in aging and age-related disease'

[47]   Jergović and Nikolich-Žugich, 'Impact of CMV upon immune aging: Facts and fiction'

[48]   Ebersole et al., 'Aging, inflammation, immunity and periodontal disease'

[49]   Budden et al., 'Emerging pathogenic links between microbiota and the gut–lung axis'

[50]   Vaiserman, Koliada and Marotta, 'Gut microbiota: A player in aging and a target for anti-aging intervention'

[51]   Ferrucci and Fabbri, 'Inflammageing: Chronic inflammation in ageing, cardiovascular disease, and frailty'; Franceschi and Campisi, 'Chronic inflammation (inflammaging) and its potential contribution to age-associated diseases'; Fulop et al., 'The integration of inflammaging in age-related diseases'

[52]   Kale et al., 'Role of immune cells in the removal of deleterious senescent cells'

[53]   Vatic, von Haehling and Ebner, 'Inflammatory biomarkers of frailty'

[54] Ferrucci and Fabbri, 'Inflammageing: chronic inflammation in ageing, cardiovascular disease, and frailty'; Franceschi and Campisi, 'Chronic inflammation (inflammaging) and its potential contribution to age-associated diseases'; Fulop et al., 'The integration of inflammaging in age-related diseases'

[55] Ferrucci and Fabbri, 'Inflammageing: Chronic inflammation in ageing, cardiovascular disease, and frailty'

[56] Franceschi and Campisi, 'Chronic inflammation (inflammaging) and its potential contribution to age-associated diseases'; Fulop et al., 'The integration of inflammaging in age-related diseases'

[57] Thursby and Juge, 'Introduction to the human gut microbiota'

[58] Salvucci, 'The human-microbiome superorganism and its modulation to restore health'

[59] Ley et al., 'Worlds within worlds: Evolution of the vertebrate gut microbiota'

[60] Budden et al., 'Emerging pathogenic links between microbiota and the gut–lung axis'; Shukla et al., 'Microbiome effects on immunity, health and disease in the lung'; Alemao et al., 'Impact of diet and

the bacterial microbiome on the mucous barrier and immune disorders'; Donovan et al., 'The role of microbiome and NLRP3 inflammasome in the gut and the lung'

[61] Kirk, '"Life in a germ-free world": Isolating life from the laboratory animal to the Bubble Boy'

[62] Al-Asmakh and Zadjali, 'Use of germ-free animal models in microbiota-related research'

[63] Verstraelen et al., 'Characterisation of the human uterine microbiome in non-pregnant women through deep sequencing of the V1-2 region of the 16S rRNA gene'

[64] Kennedy, King and Baldridge, 'Mouse microbiota models: Comparing germfree mice and antibiotics treatment as tools for modifying gut bacteria'

[65] Olszak et al., 'Microbial exposure during early life has persistent effects on natural killer T cell function'

[66] Kostic, Howitt and Garrett, 'Exploring host–microbiota interactions in animal models and humans'

[67] Kennedy, King and Baldridge, 'Mouse microbiota models: Comparing germ-free mice and antibiotics treatment as tools

for modifying gut bacteria'; Hernández-Chirlaque et al., 'Germ-free and antibiotic-treated mice are highly susceptible to epithelial injury in DSS colitis'

[68] Round and Mazmanian, 'The gut microbiota shapes intestinal immune responses during health and disease'

[69] Ivanov et al., 'Induction of intestinal Th17 cells by segmented filamentous bacteria'

[70] Turnbaugh et al., 'An obesity-associated gut microbiome with increased capacity for energy harvest'

[71] Ridaura et al., 'Gut microbiota from twins discordant for obesity modulate metabolism in mice'

[72] Zeevi et al., 'Personalized nutrition by prediction of glycemic responses'

[73] Thorburn, Macia and Mackay, 'Diet, metabolites, and "western-lifestyle" inflammatory diseases'

[74] Pascal et al., 'Microbiome and allergic dieases'

[75] Strayer et al., 'A classification of ecological boundaries'

[76] Westman, 'Measuring the inertia and resilience of ecosystems'

[77]   Westman, 'Measuring the inertia and resilience of ecosystems'

[78]   Turroni et al., 'Temporal dynamics of the gut microbiota in people sharing a confined environment, a 520-day ground-based space simulation, MARS500'; Johnson et al., 'Daily sampling reveals personalised diet-microbiome association in humans'; Wu et al., 'Linking long-term dietary patterns with gut microbial enterotypes'; David et al., 'Diet rapidly and reproducibly alters the human gut microbiome'

[79]   Bien, Palagani and Bozko, 'The intestinal microbiota dysbiosis and *Clostridium difficile* infection: Is there a relationship with inflammatory bowel disease?'

[80]   Delmas, '*Escherichia coli*: The good, the bad and the ugly'; Wexler, 'Bacteroides: The good, the bad, and the nitty-gritty'

[81]   Thorburn and Hansbro, 'Harnessing Regulatory T cells to suppress asthma'

[82]   Budden et al., 'Emerging pathogenic links between microbiota and the gut–lung axis'

[83]   Powell, 'Indoles from the commensal microbiota act via the AHR and IL-10 to tune the cellular composition of the colonic epithelium during aging'

[84]   Evans et al., 'Effects of dietary fibre type on blood pressure: A systematic review and meta-analysis of randomized controlled trials of healthy individuals'

[85]   Gianfredi et al., 'Rectal cancer: 20% risk reduction thanks to dietary fibre intake: Systematic review and meta-analysis'

[86]   Threapleton et al., 'Dietary fibre intake and risk of cardiovascular disease: Systematic review and meta-analysis'

[87]   Ojo et al., 'The role of dietary fibre in modulating gut microbiota dysbiosis in patients with type 2 diabetes: A systematic review and meta-analysis of randomised controlled trials'

[88]   Chen et al., 'Dietary fibre intake and risk of breast cancer: A systematic review and meta-analysis of epidemiological studies'

[89]   Makki et al., 'The impact of dietary fiber on gut microbiota in host health and disease'

[90]   De Filippo et al., 'Impact of diet in shaping gut microbiota revealed by a comparative study in children from Europe and rural Africa'

[91]   Riedel et al., 'Anti-inflammatory effects of bifidobacteria by inhibition of LPS-induced NF-κB activation'; Mortaz

et al., 'Anti-inflammatory effects of *Lactobacillus rahmnosus* and *Bifidobacterium breve* on cigarette smoke activated human macrophages'; Marietta et al., 'Suppression of inflammatory arthritis by human gut-derived *Prevotella histicola* in humanized mice'

[92]   Budden et al., 'Emerging pathogenic links between microbiota and the gut–lung axis'

[93]   Venegas et al., 'Short chain fatty acids (SCFAs)-mediated gut epithelial and immune regulation and its relevance for inflammatory bowel diseases'

[94]   Duscha et al., 'Propionic acid shapes the Multiple Sclerosis disease course by an immunomodulatory mechanism'

[95]   Prihandoko et al., 'Pathophysiological regulation of lung function by the free fatty acid receptor FFA4'

[96]   Buttó and Haller, 'Dysbiosis in intestinal inflammation: Cause or consequence'

[97]   Lau et al., 'Bridging the gap between gut microbial dysbiosis and cardiovascular diseases'

[98]   Bowerman et al., 'Disease-associated gut microbiome and metabolome changes in patients with chronic obstructive pulmonary disease'

[99] Rogers et al., 'From gut dysbiosis to altered brain function and mental illness: Mechanisms and pathways'

[100] Bowerman et al., 'Disease-associated gut microbiome and metabolome changes in patients with chronic obstructive pulmonary disease'; Ruiz-Canela et al., 'Comprehensive metabolomic profiling and incident cardiovascular disease: A systematic review'; Fitzpatrick and Young, 'Metabolomics – A novel window into inflammatory disease'

[101] Shukla et al., 'Microbiome effects on immunity, health and disease in the lung'

[102] Afshin et al., 'Health effects of dietary risks in 195 countries, 1990–2017: A systematic analysis for the Global Burden of Disease Study 2017'

[103] Sender, Guchs and Milo, 'Revised estimates for the number of human and bacteria cells in the body'

[104] Budden et al., 'Functional effects of the microbiota in chronic respiratory disease'

[105] Kamada et al., 'Control of pathogens and pathobionts by the gut microbiota'

[106]   Ha, Lam and Holmes, 'Mechanistic links between gut microbial community dynamics, microbial functions and metabolic health'; Bergman, 'Energy contributions of volatile fatty acids from the gastrointestinal tract in various species'

[107]   Conly and Stein, 'The production of menaquinones (vitamin K2) by intestinal bacteria and their role in maintaining coagulation homeostasis'; Uebanso et al., 'Functional roles of B-vitamins in the gut and gut-microbiome'; Dai et al., 'Amino acid metabolism in intestinal bacteria and its potential implications for mammalian reproduction'

[108]   Moore and Townsend, 'Temporal development of the infant gut microbiome'

[109]   Burch et al., 'Short-term improvements in diet quality in people newly diagnosed with type 2 diabetes are associated with smoking status, physical activity and body mass index: The 3D case series study'; Shang et al., 'Short term high fat diet induces obesity-enhancing changes in mouse. Gut microbiota that are partially

reversed by cessation of the high fat diet'

[110]   Solon-Biet et al., 'The ratio of macronutrients, not caloric intake, dictates cardiometabolic health, aging, and longevity in ad libitum-fed mice'; Zhen, 'Dietary pattern is associated with obesity in Chinese children and adolescents: Data from China Health and Nutrition Survey (CHNS)'; McGillicuddy, 'Long-term exposure to a high-fat diet results in the development of glucose intolerance and insulin resistance in interleukin-1 receptor 1-deficient mice'

[111]   Ha, Lam and Holmes, 'Mechanistic links between gut microbial community dynamics, microbial functions and metabolic health'

[112]   Peterson et al., 'Metagenomic approaches for defining the pathogenesis of inflammatory bowel diseases'

[113]   Ha, Lam and Holmes, 'Mechanistic links between gut microbial community dynamics, microbial functions and metabolic health'; Zechner, 'Inflammatory disease caused by intestinal pathobionts'; Lamont, Koo

and Hajishengallis, 'The oral microbiota: dynamic communities and host interactions'

[114] Wan et al., 'Effects of dietary fat on gut microbiota and faecal metabolites, and their relationship with cardiometabolic risk factors: A 6-month randomised controlled-feeding trial'

[115] Lecomte et al., 'Changes in gut microbiota in rats fed a high-fat diet correlate with obesity-associated metabolic parameters'; Caesar et al., 'Crosstalk between gut microbiota and dietary lipids aggravates WAT inflammation through TLR signaling'

[116] Chen et al., 'Modest sodium reduction increases circulating short-chain fatty acids in untreated hypertensives: A randomized, double-blind, placebo-controlled trial'

[117] Chen et al., 'Modest sodium reduction increases circulating short-chain fatty acids in untreated hypertensives: A randomized, double-blind, placebo-controlled trial'

[118] Wilck et al., 'Salt-responsive gut commensal modulates T H 17 axis and disease'

[119]   Holmes et al., 'Diet-microbiome interactions in health are controlled by intestinal nitrogen source constraints'

[120]   Holmes et al., 'Diet-microbiome interactions in health are controlled by intestinal nitrogen source constraints'

[121]   Holmes et al., 'Diet-microbiome interactions in health are controlled by intestinal nitrogen source constraints'

[122]   Turnbaugh et al., 'An obesity-associated gut microbiome with increased capacity for energy harvest'; Ley et al., 'Obesity alters gut microbial ecology'

[123]   Holmes et al., 'Diet-microbiome interactions in health are controlled by intestinal nitrogen source constraints'

[124]   Cox, 'Calorie restriction slows age-related microbiota changes in an Alzheimer's disease model in female mice'

[125]   Holmes et al., 'Diet-microbiome interactions in health are controlled by intestinal nitrogen source constraints'

[126]   Thaiss et al., 'Persistent microbiome alterations modulate the rate of post-dieting weight regain'

[127]   Alemao et al., 'Impact of diet and the bacterial microbiome on the mucous barrier and immune disorders'

[128]   Kostovcikova et al., 'Diet rich in animal protein promotes pro-inflammatory macrophage response and exacerbates colitis in mice'; Raimondi et al., 'Identification of mucin degraders of the human gut microbiota'

[129]   Lam et al., 'Effects of dietary fat profile on gut permeability and microbiota and their relationships with metabolic changes in mice'; Raimondi et al., 'Identification of mucin degraders of the human gut microbiota'; Gibson and Roberfroid, 'Dietary modulation of the human colonic microbiota: Introducing the concept of prebiotics'

[130]   Michalovich et al., 'Obesity and disease severity magnify disturbed microbiome-immune interactions in asthma patients'

[131]   Singh et al., 'Influence of diet on the gut microbiome and implications for human health'

[132]   Micha, Wallace and Mozaffarian, 'Red and processed meat consumption and risk of incident coronary heart disease, stroke, and diabetes mellitus: A systematic review and meta-analysis'

[133]   Mu et al., 'The colonic microbiome and epithelial transcriptome are altered

in rats fed a high-protein diet compared with a normal-protein diet'

[134] Ardalan et al., 'Dietary fat and the faecal microbiome: Where collinearity may lead to incorrect attribution of effects to fat'

[135] Groves, 'Sucrose vs glucose vs fructose: What's the difference?'

[136] Alemao et al., 'Impact of diet and the bacterial microbiome on the mucous barrier and immune disorders'

[137] Duncan, Carey-Ewend and Vaishnava, 'Spatial analysis of gut microbiome reveals a distinct ecological niche associated with the mucus layer'

[138] Beli et al., 'Restructuring of the gut microbiome by intermittent fasting precents retinopathy and prolongs survival in db/db mice'; Catterson et al., 'Short-term, intermittent fasting induces long-lasting gut health and TORindependent lifespan extension'

[139] Wahnschaffe et al., 'Predictors of clinical response to gluten-free diet in patients diagnosed with diarrhea-predominant irritable bowel syndrome'; Salas-Salvadó et al. 'Reduction in the incidence of type 2 diabetes with the Mediterranean diet:

results of the PREDIMED-Reus nutrition intervention randomized trial'

[140] WHO, 'Global health estimates 2020: Deaths by cause, age, sex, by country and by region, 2000–2019'

[141] Pfizer, 'Inflammatory bowel disease'

[142] Dicker et al., 'Global, regional, and national age-sex-specific mortality and life expectancy, 1950–2017: A systematic analysis for the Global Burden of Disease Study 2017'; Ritchie and Roser, 'Causes of death'

[143] Carto, Shannon et al., 'Out of Africa and into an ice age: On the role of global climate change in the late Pleistocene migration of early modern humans out of Africa'

[144] Diamond and Bellwood, 'Farmers and their languages: The first expansions'

[145] Armelagos, 'Brain evolution, the determinates of food choice, and the omnivore's dilemma'

[146] Leinbach et al., 'Asia'

[147] Grigg, 'Mediterranean agriculture'

[148] Grigg, 'Mixed farming in Western Europe and North America'

[149] Whittlesey, 'Fixation of shifting cultivation'; Whittlesey, 'Major agricultural regions of the earth'

[150] Yates, 'Food, land and manpower in Western Europe'; Yates, "Food production in Western Europe: An economic survey of agriculture in six countries'

[151] Wells, 'Recent economic changes: And their effect on the production and distribution of wealth and the well-being of society'

[152] Cena and Calder, 'Defining a healthy diet: Evidence for the role of contemporary dietary patterns in health and disease'; Vaughan et al., 'COPD and the gut–lung axis: The therapeutic potential of fibre'

[153] Clinton, Giovannucci and Hursting, 'The World Cancer Research Fund/American Institute for Cancer Research third expert report on diet, nutrition, physical activity, and cancer: Impact and future directions'

[154] Mozaffarian, 'Dietary and policy priorities for cardiovascular disease, diabetes, and obesity: A comprehensive review'

[155] Cordain et al., 'Origins and evolution of the Western diet: Health implications for the 21st century'

[156]   The Global Asthma Network, 'The global asthma report 2018'

[157]   Australian Institute of Health and Welfare, 'Mortality from asthma and COPD in Australia'

[158]   Wood, 'Diet, obesity, and asthma'

[159]   ABS, 'Australian health survey: Consumption of food groups from the australian dietary guidelines, 2011-12'

[160]   'WHO, 'Obesity and overweight'

[161]   Australian Institute of Health and Welfare, 'Overweight and obesity: An interactive insight'

[162]   Hales et al., 'Prevalence of obesity among adults and youth: United States, 2015-2016'

[163]   Beuther and Sutherland, 'Overweight, obesity, and incident asthma: A metaanalysis of prospective epidemiologic studies'

[164]   Wood, 'Diet, obesity, and asthma'

[165]   Wood, Garg and Gibson, 'A high-fat challenge increases airway inflammation and impairs bronchodilator recovery in asthma'

[166]   Halnes et al., 'Soluble fibre meal challenge reduces airway inflammation and expression of GPR43 and GPR41 in asthma'

[167]   McLoughlin et al., 'Soluble fibre supplementation with and without a probiotic in adults with asthma: A 7-day randomised, double blind, three way cross-over trial'

[168]   Wood et al., 'Lycopene-rich treatments modify noneosinophilic airway inflammation in asthma: proof of concept'

[169]   Wood et al., 'Manipulating antioxidant intake in asthma: A randomized controlled trial'

[170]   National Asthma Council, 'Healthy eating for asthma'; Global Initiative for Asthma, 'Global strategy for asthma management and prevention (2019 update)'

[171]   Bucci, 'Transfer of host phenotypes through microbiota transplantation'

[172]   Zhang et al., 'Impact of fecal microbiota transplantation on obesity and metabolic syndrome: A systematic review'; Infectious Diseases Society of America, 'Rapid and unexpected weight gain after fecal transplant'

[173]   Well+Good Editors, '5 ways to support brain health, according to a neuroscientist'

[174]   Tapia Granados and Diez Roux, 'Life and death during the Great Depression'

[175]   Kirkpatrick, 'Do DNA-based diets work?'

[176]   Fricker, Deane and Hansbro, 'Animal models of chronic obstructive pulmonary disease'; Jones et al., 'Animal models of COPD: What do they tell us?'

[177]   Keely, Talley and Hansbro, 'Pulmonary-intestinal cross-talk in mucosal inflammatory disease'; Budden et al., 'Emerging pathogenic links between microbiota and the gut–lung axis'; Shukla et al., 'Microbiome effects on immunity, health and disease in the lung'

[178]   Microba, 'Gut microbe testing and analysis Australia'

[179]   Stanford et al., 'Associations among plant-based diet quality, uremic toxins, and gut microbiota profile in adults undergoing hemodialysis therapy'

[180]   Bauer, 'What is the Okinawa diet?'

[181]   Gunnars and Link, 'Mediterranean diet 101: A meal plan and beginner's guide'

[182]   Okinawa Research Center for Longevity Science, 'About'

[183]   Gerber   and   Hoffman,   'The
         Mediterranean diet: health, science and
         society'

[184]   Tang et al., 'Administration of a
         probiotic   with   peanut   oral
         immunotherapy: A randomized trial'

[185]   Tan et al., 'The role of short-chain
         fatty acids in health and disease'

[186]   Evans, 'Dietary fibre and cardiovascular
         health: a review of current evidence
         and policy'

[187]   Diep, Baranowski and Baranowski, 'The
         impact of fruit and vegetable intake on
         weight management'

[188]   Pérez-Jiménez et al., 'Identification of
         the 100 richest dietary sources of
         polyphenols: An application of the
         Phenol-Explorer database'

[189]   Singh et al., 'Beneficial Effects of
         Dietary Polyphenols on Gut Microbiota
         and Strategies to Improve Delivery
         Efficiency'

[190]   Singh et al., 'Influence of diet on the
         gut microbiome and implications for
         human health'

[191]   Dagfinn et al., 'Whole grain
         consumption and risk of cardiovascular
         disease, cancer, and all cause and cause
         specific mortality: Systematic review

and dose-response meta-analysis of prospective studies'

[192] Rossi et al., 'Dietary protein-fiber ratio associates with circulating levels of indoxyl sulfate and p-cresyl sulfate in chronic kidney disease patients'

[193] Roach et al., 'Improved plasma lipids, anti-inflammatory activity, and microbiome shifts in overweight participants: Two clinical studies on oral supplementation with algal sulfated polysaccharide'

[194] Ghosh et al., 'Mediterranean diet intervention alters the gut microbiome in older people reducing frailty and improving health status: The NU-AGE 1-year dietary intervention across five European countries'

[195] Wolters et al., 'Dietary fat, the gut microbiota, and metabolic health – A systematic review conducted within the MyNewGut project'

[196] Watson et al., 'A randomised trial of the effect of omega-3 polyunsaturated fatty acid supplements on the human intestinal microbiota'

[197] Wan et al., 'Effects of dietary fat on gut microbiota and faecal metabolites, and their relationship with

cardiometabolic risk factors: A 6-month randomised controlled-feeding trial'

[198]   Patridge et al., 'Food additives: Assessing the impact of exposure to permitted emulsifiers on bowel and metabolic health – introducing the FADiets study'

[199]   Ruiz-Ojeda et al., 'Effects of sweeteners on the gut microbiota: A review of experimental studies and clinical trials'

[200]   Goel, Sharma and Garg, 'Effect of alcohol consumption on cardiovascular health'

[201]   Yang and Eun, 'Fermentation and sensory characteristics of korean traditional fermented liquor (makgeolli) added with citron (citrus junos SIEB ex TANAKA) juice'

[202]   Corliss, 'Is red wine actually good for your heart?'; Mayo Clinic, 'Red wine and resveratrol: Good for your heart?'

[203]   Collins, 'How to cook your vegies to maintain good nutrition and support your immune system during coronavirus'

References

Afshin, Ashkan et al. 'Health effects of dietary risks in 195 countries, 1990–2017: A systematic analysis for the Global Burden of Disease Study 2017'. https://doi.org/10.1016/S0140-6736(19)300 41-8.

Al-Asmakh, Maha and Zadjali, Fahad. 'Use of germ-free animal models in microbiota-related research'. https://doi.org/10.4014/jmb.1501.01039.

Alatab, Sudabeh et al. 'The global, regional, and national burden of inflammatory bowel disease in 195 countries and territories, 1990–2017: A systematic analysis for the Global Burden of Disease Study 2017'. https://www.thelancet.com/journals/langas/article/PIIS2468-1253(19)30333-4/f ulltext.

Alemao, Charlotte A. et al. 'Impact of diet and the bacterial microbiome on the mucous barrier and immune disorders'. https://doi.org/10.1111/a ll.14548.

Allan, G. Michael and Aaroll, Bruce. 'Prevention and treatment of the common cold: Making sense of the evidence'. https://www.ncbi.nlm.nih .gov/pmc/articles/PMC3928210/.

American Academy of Allergy Asthma and Immunology ('AAAAI'). 'Atopic March defined'. https://www.aaaai.org/Tools-for-the-Public/Allergy ,-Asthma-Immunology-Glossary/Atopic-March-De fined.

American Autoimmune Related Diseases Association ('AARDA') and National Coalition of Autoimmune Patient Groups ('NCAPG'). 'The cost burden of autoimmune disease: The latest front in the war on healthcare spending'. http:/ /www.diabetesed.net/page/_files/autoimmune-dise ases.pdf.

Ardalan, Zaid S. et al. 'Dietary fat and the faecal microbiome: Where collinearity may lead to incorrect attribution of effects to fat'. http://dx. doi.org/10.1136/gutjnl-2019-319628.

Aristizábal, Beatriz and González, Ángel. 'Innate immune system'. https://www.ncbi.nlm.nih.gov/bo oks/NBK459455/

Armanios, Mary et al. 'Translational strategies in aging and age-related disease'. https://doi.org/10. 1038/nm.4004.

Armelagos, George J. 'Brain evolution, the determinates of food choice, and the omnivore's dilemma'. https://doi.org/10.1080/10408398.2011. 63 5817.

Asrani, Sumeet K et al. 'Burden of liver diseases in the world'. https://pubmed.ncbi.nlm.nih.gov/30 266282/.

Australian Bureau of Statistics ('ABS'). 'Australian health survey: Consumption of food groups from the australian dietary guidelines, 2011-12'. https ://www.abs.gov.au/AUSSTATS/abs@.nsf/Lookup/4 364.0.55.012.

Australian Bureau of Statistics ('ABS'). 'Australian health survey: Nutrition first results – foods and nutrients'. https://www.abs.gov.au/statistics/health /health-conditions-and-risks/australian-health-surv eynutrition-first-results-foods-and-nutrients/latest -release.

Australian Institute of Health and Welfare. 'Mortality from asthma and COPD in Australia'. https://www.aihw.gov.au/reports/chronicrespirato ry-conditions/mortality-from-asthma-and-copd-in-australia/summary.

Australian Institute of Health and Welfare. 'Overweight and obesity: an interactive insight'. https://www.aihw.gov.au/reports/overweightobesi ty/overweight-and-obesity-an-interactive-insight/c ontents/whatis-overweight-and-obesity.

Bauer, Shannon. 'What is the Okinawa diet?'. ht tps://web.archive.org/web/20210614004201/https: //www.shape.com/healthy-eating/diettips/okinawa-diet.

Beli, Eleni et al. 'Restructuring of the gut microbiome by intermittent fasting precents retinopathy and prolongs survival in db/db mice'. https://doi.org/10.2337/db18-0158.

Bergman, E.N. 'Energy contributions of volatile fatty acids from the gastrointestinal tract in various species'. https://doi.org/10.1152/physrev.1990.70.2.567.

Better Health Channel. 'Pelvic inflammatory disease (PID)'. https://www.betterhealth.vic.gov.a u/health/healthyliving/pelvic-inflammatorydisease-p id.

Beuther, David A. and Sutherland E.R. 'Overweight, obesity, and incident asthma: a meta-analysis of prospective epidemiologic studies'. https://doi.org/10.1164/rccm.200611-171 7oc.

Bien, Justyna, Palagani, Vindhya and Bozko, Przemyslaw. 'The intestinal microbiota dysbiosis and Clostridium difficile infection: Is there a relationship with inflammatory bowel disease?' https://doi.org/10.1177/1756283X12454590.

Bilaver, Lucy A et al. 'Economic burden of food allergy: A systematic review.' https://www.annallergy.org/article/S1081-1206(19)30051-1/fulltext.

Bowerman, Kate L. et al. 'Disease-associated gut microbiome and metabolome changes in patients with chronic obstructive pulmonary disease'. https://doi.org/10.1038/s41467-020-19701-0.

Bowerman, Kate L. et al. 'Disease-associated gut microbiome and metabolome changes in patients with chronic obstructive pulmonary disease'. https://doi.org/10.1038/s41467-020-19701-0.

Bucci, Mirella. 'Transfer of host phenotypes through microbiota transplantation'. https://www.nature.com/articles/d42859-019-00016-0.

Budden, Kurtis F. et al. 'Emerging pathogenic links between microbiota and the gut–lung axis'. https://doi.org/10.1038/nrmicro.2016.142.

Budden, Kurtis F. et al. 'Functional effects of the microbiota in chronic respiratory disease'. https://doi.org/10.1016/s2213-2600(18)30510-1.

Burch, Emily et al. 'Short-term improvements in diet quality in people newly diagnosed with type 2 diabetes are associated with smoking status, physical activity and body mass index: The 3D case series study'. https://doi.org/10.1038/s41387-020-0128-3.

Buttó, Ludovica F. and Haller, Dirk. 'Dysbiosis in intestinal inflammation: Cause or consequence'. https://doi.org/10.1016/j.ijmm.2016.02.010.

Caesar, Robert et al. 'Crosstalk between gut microbiota and dietary lipids aggravates WAT inflammation through TLR signaling'. https://doi.org/10.1016/j.cmet.2015.07.026.

Caggiu, Elisa et al. 'Inflammation, infectious triggers, and Parkinson's disease'. https://www.frontiersin.org/articles/10.3389/fneur.2019.00122/full.

Cancer Treatment Centers of America ('CTCA'). 'Inflammation linked to cancer, but lifestyle changes may help'. https://www.cancercenter.co m/community/blog/2018/08/inflammation-linked-t o-cancer-butlifestyle-changes-may-help.

Carto, Shannon et al. 'Out of Africa and into an ice age: On the role of global climate change in the late Pleistocene migration of early modern humans out of Africa'. https://doi.org/10.1016/j.j hevol.2008.09.004.

Catterson, James H. et al. 'Short-term, intermittent fasting induces long-lasting gut health and TOR-independent lifespan extension'. https: //doi.org/10.1016/j.cub.2018.04.015.

Cena, Hellas and Calder, Phillip C. 'Defining a healthy diet: Evidence for the role of contemporary dietary patterns in health and disease'. https://doi.org/10.3390%2Fnu12020334.

Centres for Disease Control and Prevention ('CDC'). 'Stroke signs and symptoms'. https://w ww.cdc.gov/stroke/signs_symptoms.htm.

Chen, Li et al. 'Modest sodium reduction increases circulating Short-Chain Fatty Acids in untreated hypertensives: A randomized,

double-blind, placebo-controlled trial'. https://do
i.org/10.1161/hypertensionaha.120.14800.

Chen, Sumei et al. 'Dietary fibre intake and risk
of breast cancer: A systematic review and
meta-analysis of epidemiological studies'. https://
doi.org/10.18632%2Foncotarget.13140.

Clinton, Steven K., Giovannucci, Edward L. and
Hursting, Stephen D. 'The World Cancer
Research Fund/American Institute for Cancer
Research Third Expert Report on diet, nutrition,
physical activity, and cancer: Impact and future
directions'. https://doi.org/10.1093/jn/nxz268.

Collins, Clare. 'How to cook your vegies to
maintain good nutrition and support your
immune system during coronavirus'. https://ww
w.abc.net.au/news/science/2020-04-13/cooking-ve
getables-for-bestnutrition-during-coronavirus/120
59854.

Conly, J.M. and Stein, K. 'The production of
menaquinones (vitamin K2) by intestinal bacteria
and their role in maintaining coagulation
homeostasis'. https://pubmed.ncbi.nlm.nih.gov/149
2156/.

Cordain, Loren et al. 'Origins and evolution of the Western diet: Health implications for the 21st century'. https://doi.org/10.1093/ajcn.81.2.341.

Corliss, Julie. 'Is red wine actually good for your heart?'. https://www.health.harvard.edu/blog/is-red-wine-good-actually-for-yourheart-2018021913285.

Cox, Laura M. et al. 'Calorie restriction slows age-related microbiota changes in an Alzheimer's disease model in female mice'. https://doi.org/10.1038/s41598-019-54187-x.

Dadonaite, Bernadeta and Roser, Max. 'Pneumonia'. https://ourworldindata.org/pneumonia#why-are-children-dying-from-pneumonia.

Dagfinn, Aune et al. 'Whole grain consumption and risk of cardiovascular disease, cancer, and all cause and cause specific mortality: Systematic review and dose-response meta-analysis of prospective studies'. https://doi.org/10.1136%2Fbmj.i2716.

Dai, Zhaolai et al. 'Amino acid metabolism in intestinal bacteria and its potential implications for mammalian reproduction'. https://doi.org/10.1093/molehr/gav003.

David, Lawrence A. et al. 'Diet rapidly and reproducibly alters the human gut microbiome'. https://doi.org/10.1038/nature12820.

Davita Kidney Care. 'Anemia and chronic kidney disease.' https://www.davita.com/education/kidney-disease/risk-factors/anemia-andchronic-kidney-disease.

De Filippo, Carlotta et al. 'Impact of diet in shaping gut microbiota revealed by a comparative study in children from Europe and rural Africa'. https://doi.org/10.1073/pnas.1005963107.

Delmas, Julien. 'Escherichia coli: The good, the bad and the ugly'. http://dx.doi.org/10.4172/2327-5073.1000195.

Diamond, Jared and Bellwood, Peter. 'Farmers and their languages: The first expansions'. https://doi.org/10.1126/science.1078208.

Dicker, Daniel et al. 'Global, regional, and national age-sex-specific mortality and life expectancy, 1950–2017: A systematic analysis for the Global Burden of Disease Study 2017'. https://www.the

lancet.com/journals/lancet/article/PIIS0140-6736(1 8)31891-9/fulltext.

Diep, C.S., Baranowski, J and Baranowski, T. 'The impact of fruit and vegetable intake on weight management'. https://doi.org/10.1533/978178242 0996.2.59.

Dinet, Virginie et al. 'Brain–immune interactions and neuroinflammation after traumatic brain injury'. https://www.frontiersin.org/articles/10.338 9/fnins.2019.01178/full.

Donovan, C. et al. 'The role of microbiome and NLRP3 inflammasome in the gut and the lung'. https://doi.org/10.1002/JLB.3MR0720-472RR.

Duncan, Kellyanne, Carey-Ewend, Kelly and Vaishnava, Shipra. 'Spatial analysis of gut microbiome reveals a distinct ecological niche associated with the mucus layer'. https://doi.org /10.1080/19490976.2021.1874815.

Duscha, Alexander et al. 'Propionic acid shapes the Multiple Sclerosis disease course by an immunomodulatory mechanism'. https://doi.org/1 0.1016/j.cell.2020.02.035.

Ebersole, Jeffery L. et al. 'Aging, inflammation, immunity and periodontal disease'. https://doi.or g/10.1111/prd.12135.

European Respiratory Society ('ERS'). 'The economic burden of lung disease'. https://www. erswhitebook.org/chapters/the-economicburden-of-lung-disease/.

Evans, Charlotte E.L. et al. 'Effects of dietary fibre type on blood pressure: a systematic review and meta-analysis of randomized controlled trials of healthy individuals'. https://doi.org/10.1097/HJH.0 00000000000000515.

Evans, Charlotte E.L. 'Dietary fibre and cardiovascular health: a review of current evidence and policy'. https://doi.org/10.1017/s00 29665119000673.

Feigin, Valery L et al. 'Global, regional, and national burden of neurological disorders, 1990–2016: A systematic analysis for the Global Burden of Disease Study 2016'. https://www.the lancet.com/journals/laneur/article/PIIS1474-4422(1 8)30499-X/fulltext.

Ferrucci, Luigi and Fabbri, Elisa. 'Inflammageing: chronic inflammation in ageing, cardiovascular disease, and frailty'. https://doi.org/10.1038/s415 69-018-0064-2.

Fitzpatrick, Martin and Young, Stephen P. 'Metabolomics – A novel window into inflammatory disease'. https://doi.org/10.4414%2F smw.2013.13743.

Franceschi, Claudio and Campisi, Judith. 'Chronic inflammation (inflammaging) and its potential contribution to age-associated diseases'. https:// doi.org/10.1093/gerona/glu057.

Fricker, Michael, Deane, Andrew and Hansbro, Phillip M. 'Animal models of chronic obstructive pulmonary disease'. https://doi.org/10.1517/17 4 60441.2014.909805.

Fulop, Tamas et al. 'The integration of inflammaging in age-related diseases'. https://doi. org/10.1016/j.smim.2018.09.003.

Gerber, Mariette and Hoffman, Richard. 'The Mediterranean diet: health, science and society'. https://doi.org/10.1017/s0007114514003912.

Ghosh, T.S. et al. 'Mediterranean diet intervention alters the gut microbiome in older people reducing frailty and improving health status: the

NU-AGE 1-year dietary intervention across five European countries'. https://doi.org/10.1136/gutj nl-2019-319654.

Gianfredi, Vincenza et al. 'Rectal cancer: 20% risk reduction thanks to dietary fibre intake. Systematic review and meta-analysis'. https://doi .org/10.3390/nu11071579.

Gibson, G.R. and Roberfroid, M.B. 'Dietary modulation of the human colonic microbiota: Introducing the concept of prebiotics'. https://d oi.org/10.1093/jn/125.6.1401.

Global Initiative for Asthma. 'Global strategy for asthma management and prevention (2019 update)'. https://ginasthma.org/wp-content/upload s/2019/06/GINA-2019-main-report-June-2019-wm s.pdf.

Goel, Sunny, Sharma, Abhishek and Garg, Aakash. 'Effect of alcohol consumption on cardiovascular health'. https://doi.org/10.1007/s11886-018-0962-2.

Grigg, D.B. 'Mediterranean agriculture'. The Agricultural Systems of the World: An Evolutionary Approach. Cambridge University Press (1974).

Grigg, D.B. 'Mixed farming in Western Europe and North America'. The Agricultural Systems of the World: An Evolutionary Approach. Cambridge University Press (1974).

Groves, Melissa. 'Sucrose vs Glucose vs Fructose: What's the difference?'. https://www.healthline.com/nutrition/sucrose-glucose-fructose.

Gunnars, Kris and Link, Rachael. 'Mediterranean diet 101: A meal plan and beginner's guide'. https://www.healthline.com/nutrition/mediterranean-diet-meal-plan.

Ha, Connie WY., Lam, Yan Y. and Holmes, Andrew J. 'Mechanistic links between gut microbial community dynamics, microbial functions and metabolic health'. https://doi.org/10.3748%2Fwjg.v20.i44.16498

Hales, Craig M. et al. 'Prevalence of obesity among adults and youth: United States, 2015-2016'. https://www.cdc.gov/nchs/products/databriefs/db288.htm.

Halnes, Isabel et al. 'Soluble fibre meal challenge reduces airway inflammation and expression of GPR43 and GPR41 in asthma'. https://doi.org/10.3390%2Fnu9010057.

Hirode, Grishma et al. 'Trends in the burden of chronic liver disease among hospitalized US adults'. https://jamanetwork.com/journals/jamanetworkopen/fullarticle/2763783.

Healthgrades. 'Liver failure'. https://www.healthgrades.com/right-care/liverconditions/liver-failure.

Hernández-Chirlaque, Cristina et al. 'Germ-free and antibiotic-treated mice are highly susceptible to epithelial injury in DSS Colitis'. https://doi.org/10.1093/ecco-jcc/jjw096.

Hoffman, Matthew. 'Autoimmune disorders?' https://www.webmd.com/ato-z-guides/autoimmune-diseases.

Holmes, Andrew J. et al. 'Diet-microbiome interactions in health are controlled by intestinal nitrogen source constraints'. https://doi.org/10.1016/j.cmet.2016.10.021.

Hur, Ji-Yeun et al. 'The innate immunity protein IFITM3 modulates γ-secretase in Alzheimer's disease'. https://www.nature.com/articles/s41586-020-2681-2.

Infectious Diseases Society of America. 'Rapid and unexpected weight gain after fecal

transplant'. https://www.sciencedaily.com/releases
/2015/02/150204125810.htm.

Ivanov, Ivaylo I. et. al. 'Induction of intestinal
Th17 cells by segmented filamentous bacteria'.
https://doi.org/10.1016%2Fj. cell.2009.09.033.

Jacka, Felice N. et al. 'A randomised controlled
trial of dietary improvement for adults with
major depression (the 'SMILES' trial)'. https://do
i.org/10.1186/s12916-017-0791-y

Jean, Tiffany. 'Allergic rhintis'. https://www.medsc
ape.com/answers/134825-4365/what-is-the-econo
mic-burden-of-allergicrhinitis-hay-fever.

Jergović, Mladen, Contreras, Nico A. and
Nikolich-Žugich, Janko. 'Impact of CMV upon
immune aging: Facts and fiction'. https://doi.org/
10.1007/s00430-019-00605-w.

Johnson, Abigail J. et al. 'Daily sampling reveals
personalized diet-microbiome associations in
humans'. https://doi.org/10.1016/j.chom.2019.05.0
05.

Jones, Bernadette et al. 'Animal models of COPD:
What do they tell us?'. https://doi.org/10.1111/r
esp.12908.

Kale, Abhijit et al. 'Role of immune cells in the removal of deleterious senescent cells'. https://doi.org/10.1186/s12979-020-00187-9.

Kamada, Nobuhiko et al. 'Control of pathogens and pathobionts by the gut microbiota'. https://doi.org/10.1038/ni.2608.

Keely, S., Talley, N.J. and Hansbro, P.M. 'Pulmonary-intestinal cross-talk in mucosal inflammatory disease'. https://doi.org/10.1038/mi.2011.55.

Kennedy, Elizabeth A., King, Katherine Y. and Baldridge, Megan T. 'Mouse microbiota models: Comparing germ-free mice and antibiotics treatment as tools for modifying gut bacteria'. https://doi.org/10.3389/fphys.2018.01534.

Kirk, Robert G.W. '"Life in a germ-free world": Isolating Life from the Laboratory Animal to the Bubble Boy'. https://doi.org/10.1353%2Fbhm.2012.0028.

Kirkpatrick, Kristin. 'Do DNA-based diets work?'. https://www.today.com/health/do-personalized-diets-work-t183387.

Kostic, Aleksandar D., Howitt, Michael R. and Garrett, Wendy S. 'Exploring host–microbiota interactions in animal models and humans'. http://www.genesdev.org/cgi/doi/10.1101/gad.212522.112.

Kostovcikova, Klara et al. 'Diet rich in animal protein promotes pro-inflammatory macrophage response and exacerbates colitis in mice'. https://doi.org/10.3389/fimmu.2019.00919.

Lam, Yan Y. et al. 'Effects of dietary fat profile on gut permeability and microbiota and their relationships with metabolic changes in mice'. https://doi.org/10.1002/oby.21122.

Lamont, Richard J., Koo, Hyun and Hajishengallis, George. 'The oral microbiota: dynamic communities and host interactions'. https://doi.org/10.1038/s41579-018-0089-x.

Lau, Kimberley et al. 'Bridging the gap between gut microbial dysbiosis and cardiovascular diseases'. https://doi.org/10.3390/nu9080859.

Lichtenstein, Gary R et al. 'Lifetime economic burden of Crohn's Disease and Ulcerative Colitis by age at diagnosis'. https://pubmed.ncbi.nlm.nih.gov/31326606/.

Lecomte, Virginie et al. 'Changes in gut microbiota in rats fed a high fat diet correlate with obesity-associated metabolic parameters'. https://doi.org/10.1371/journal.pone.0126931.

Leinbach, Thomas R. et al. 'Asia'. https://www.britannica.com/place/Asia.

Ley, Ruth E. et al. 'Obesity alters gut microbial ecology'. https://doi.org/10.1073/pnas.0504978102.

Ley, Ruth E. et al. 'Worlds within worlds: evolution of the vertebrate gut microbiota'. https://doi.org/10.1038/nrmicro1978.

López-Otín, Carlos et al. 'The hallmarks of aging'. https://doi.org/10.1016/j.cell.2013.05.039.

Makki, Kassem et al. 'The impact of dietary fiber on gut microbiota in host health and disease'. https://doi.org/10.1016/j. chom.2018.05.012.

Marietta, Eric V. et al. 'Suppression of inflammatory arthritis by human gut-derived Prevotella histicola in humanized mice'. https://onlinelibrary.wiley.com/doi/full/10.1002/art.39785.

Mayo Clinic. 'Inflammatory bowel disease (IBD)'. https://www.mayoclinic.org/diseases-conditions/in flammatory-bowel-disease/symptomscauses/syc-2 0353315.

Mayo Clinic. 'Red wine and resveratrol: Good for your heart?'. https://www.mayoclinic.org/dise ases-conditions/heart-disease/in-depth/red-wine/a rt-20048281.

McGillicuddy, Fiona C. et al. 'Long-term exposure to a high-fat diet results in the development of glucose intolerance and insulin resistance in interleukin-1 receptor 1-deficient mice'. https://d oi.org/10.1152/ajpendo.00297.2013.

McLoughlin, Rebecca et al. 'Soluble fibre supplementation with and without a probiotic in adults with asthma: A 7-day randomised, double blind, three way cross-over trial'. https:/ /doi.org/10.1016/j.ebiom.2019.07.048.

Micha, Renata, Wallace, Sarah K. and Mozaffarian, Dariush. 'Red and processed meat consumption and risk of incident coronary heart disease, stroke, and diabetes mellitus: a systematic review and metaanalysis'. https://doi.org/10.1161/circulat ionaha.109.924977.

Michalovich, David et al. 'Obesity and disease severity magnify disturbed microbiome-immune interactions in asthma patients'. https://doi.org/10.1038/s41467-019-13751-9.

Microba. 'Gut microbe testing and analysis Australia'. https://insight.microba.com/.

Mindgardens Neuroscience Network ('Mindgardens'). 'Review of the burden of disease for neurological, mental health and substance use disorders in Australia'. https://www.neura.edu.au/wp-content/uploads/2019/03/MINDGARDENS-WHITE-PAPER-FINAL-14th-March-2019.pdf.

Moore, Rebecca E. and Townsend, Steven D. 'Temporal development of the infant gut microbiome'. https://doi.org/10.1098/rsob.190128.

Mortaz, Esmaeil et al. 'Anti-inflammatory effects of Lactobacillus Rahmnosus and Bifidobacterium Breve on cigarette smoke activated human macrophages'. https://doi.org/10.1371/journal.pone.0136455.

Mozaffarian, Dariush. 'Dietary and policy priorities for cardiovascular disease, diabetes, and obesity: a comprehensive review'. https://doi.org/10.1161/circulationaha.115.018585.

Mu, Chunlong et al. 'The colonic microbiome and epithelial transcriptome are altered in rats fed a high-protein diet compared with a normal-protein diet'. https://doi.org/10.3945/jn.115.223990.

National Asthma Council. 'Healthy eating for asthma'. https://www.asthmahandbook.org.au/clinical-issues/food/healthy-eating.

National Cancer Institute. 'Symptoms of cancer'. https://www.cancer.gov/about-cancer/diagnosis-staging/symptoms.

National Kidney Foundation. 'Global facts: About kidney disease'. https://www.kidney.org/kidneydisease/global-facts-about-kidney-disease.

Njagi, Purity et al. 'Economic costs of infertility care for patients in low-income and middle-income countries: a systematic review protocol'. https://bmjopen.bmj.com/content/10/11/e042951.

Nunes, Carlos, Pereira, Ana M. and Morais-Almeida. 'Asthma costs and social impact'. https://doi.org/10.1186%2Fs40733-016-0029-3.

Ojo, Omorogieva et al. 'The role of dietary fibre in modulating gut microbiota dysbiosis in patients with Type 2 Diabetes: a systematic review and meta-analysis of randomised controlled trials'. https://doi.org/10.3390/nu12113239.

Okinawa Research Center for Longevity Science. 'About'. https://orcls.org/about/.

Olszak, Torsten et al. 'Microbial exposure during early life has persistent effects on natural killer T cell function'. https://doi.org/10.1126/science.1219328.

Pascal, Mariona et al. 'Microbiome and allergic dieases'. https://doi.org/10.3389%2Ffimmu.2018.01584.

Patridge, D. et al. 'Food additives: Assessing the impact of exposure to permitted emulsifiers on bowel and metabolic health – introducing the FADiets study'. https://doi.org/10.1111/nbu.12408.

Pérez-Jiménez, J. et al. 'Identification of the 100 richest dietary sources of polyphenols: an application of the Phenol-Explorer database'. https://www.nature.com/articles/ejcn2010221.

Peterson, Daniel A. et al. 'Metagenomic approaches for defining the pathogenesis of inflammatory bowel diseases'. https://doi.org/10.1016%2Fj.chom.2008.05.001.

Pfizer. 'Inflammatory bowel disease'. https://web.archive.org/web/20220120040553/https://www.pfizer.com/news/featured_stories/featured_stories_detail/inflammatory_bowel_disease.

Powell, Domonica N. et al. 'Indoles from the commensal microbiota act via the AHR and IL-10 to tune the cellular composition of the colonic epithelium during aging'. https://doi.org/10.1073/pnas.2003004117/

Prihandoko, Rudi et al. 'Pathophysiological regulation of lung function by the free fatty acid receptor FFA4'. https://doi.org/10.1126/scitranslmed.aaw9009.

Puac, Sanela. '25 noteworthy allergy statistics & facts to know in 2022'. https://medalerthelp.org/blog/allergy-statistics/.

Raimondi, Stefano et al. 'Identification of mucin degraders of the human gut microbiota'. https://doi.org/10.1038/s41598-021-90553-4.

Ridaura, Vanessa K. et al. 'Gut microbiota from twins discordant for obesity modulate metabolism in mice'. https://doi.org/10.1126/science.1241214.

Riedel, Christian U. et al. 'Anti-inflammatory effects of bifidobacteria by inhibition of LPS-induced NF-κB activation'. https://doi.org/10.3748%2Fwjg.v12.i23.3729.

Ritchie, Hannah and Roser, Max. 'Causes of death'. https://ourworldindata.org/causes-of-death.

Roach, Lauren A. et al. 'Improved plasma lipids, anti-inflammatory activity, and microbiome shifts in overweight participants: Two clinical studies on oral supplementation with algal sulfated polysaccharide'. https://doi.org/10.3390/md20080500.

Rogers, G.B. et al. 'From gut dysbiosis to altered brain function and mental illness: mechanisms and pathways'. https://doi.org/10.1038/mp.2016.50.

Rossi, M. et al. 'Dietary protein-fiber ratio associates with circulating levels of indoxyl sulfate and p-cresyl sulfate in chronic kidney disease

patients'. https://doi.org/10.1016/j.numecd.2015.0
3.015.

Round, June L. and Mazmanian, Sarkis K. 'The
gut microbiota shapes intestinal immune
responses during health and disease'. https://doi
.org/10.1038/nri2515.

Ruiz-Canela, Miguel et al. 'Comprehensive
metabolomic profiling and incident cardiovascular
disease: A systematic review'. https://doi.org/10.
1161/JAHA.117.005705.

Ruiz-Ojeda, Francisco J. et al. 'Effects of
sweeteners on the gut microbiota: A review of
experimental studies and clinical trials'. https://d
oi.org/10.1093/advances/nmy037.

Saad-Naguib, Michael H. et al. 'Cost-effective
analysis of infertility treatment in women with
anovulatory polycystic ovarian syndrome'. https:
//journals.lww.com/grh/Fulltext/2020/09010/Cost_
effective_analysis_of_infertility_treatment.4.aspx.

Salas-Salvadó, Jordi et al. 'Reduction in the
incidence of type 2 diabetes with the
Mediterranean diet: results of the
PREDIMED-Reus nutrition intervention

randomized trial'. https://doi.org/10.2337/dc10-1288.

Salvucci, E. 'The human-microbiome superorganism and its modulation to restore health'. https://doi.org/10.1080/09637486.2019.1580682.

Scudellari, Megan. 'To stay young, kill zombie cells'. https://doi.org/10.1038/550448a.

Sender, Ron, Fuchs, Dhai and Milo, Ron. 'Revised estimates for the number of human and bacteria cells in the body'. https://doi.org/10.1371/journal.pbio.1002533.

Sepanlou, Sadaf G. et al. 'The global, regional, and national burden of cirrhosis by cause in 195 countries and territories, 1990–2017: a systematic analysis for the Global Burden of Disease Study 2017'. https://www.thelancet.com/journals/langas/article/PIIS2468-1253(19)30349-8/fulltext.

Shang, Yue et al. 'Short term high fat diet induces obesity-enhancing changes in mouse. Gut microbiota that are partially reversed by cessation of the high fat diet'. https://doi.org/10.1007/s11745-017-4253-2.

Shukla, Shakti D. et al. 'Microbiome effects on immunity, health and disease in the lung'. https://doi.org/10.1038%2Fcti.2017.6.

Singh, Amit K. et al. 'Beneficial Effects of Dietary Polyphenols on Gut Microbiota and Strategies to Improve Delivery Efficiency'. https://doi.org/10.3390/nu11092216.

Singh, Rasnik K. et al. 'Influence of diet on the gut microbiome and implications for human health'. https://doi.org/10.1186/s12967-017-1175-y.

Solon-Biet, Samantha M. et al. 'The ratio of macronutrients, not caloric intake, dictates cardiometabolic health, aging, and longevity in ad libitum-fed mice'. https://doi.org/10.1016/j.cmet.2014.02.009.

Stanford, Jordan et al. 'Associations among plant-based diet quality, uremic toxins, and gut microbiota profile in adults undergoing hemodialysis therapy'. https://doi.org/10.1053/j.jrn.2020.07.008.

Stewart, Bernard W. and Wild, Christopher P. (eds). 'World Cancer Report 2014'. https://publ

ications.iarc.fr/Non-Series-Publications/World-Ca
ncer-Reports/World-Cancer-Report-2014.

Strayer, David L. et al. 'A classification of
ecological boundaries'. https://doi.org/10.1641/00
06-3568(2003)053[0723:ACOEB]2.0.CO;2.

Su, Junhong et al. 'Remodeling of the gut
microbiome during Ramadan-associated
intermittent fasting'. https://doi.org/10.1093/ajcn/
nqaa388.

Su, Yanfung et al. 'Tracking total spending on
tuberculosis by source and function in 135
low-income and middle-income countries,
2000–17: A financial modelling study'. https://w
ww.thelancet.com/journals/laninf/article/PIIS1473-
3099(20)30124-9/fulltext.

Sun, Hui et al. 'Global, regional, and national
prevalence and disability-adjusted life-years for
infertility in 195 countries and territories,
1990–2017: results from a global burden of
disease study, 2017'. https://www.ncbi.nlm.nih.go
v/pmc/articles/PMC6932903/.

Tan, Jian et al. 'The role of short-chain fatty acids
in health and disease'. https://doi.org/10.1016/b9
78-0-12-800100-4.00003-9.

Tang, Mimi L.K. et al., 'Administration of a probiotic with peanut oral immunotherapy: A randomized trial'. https://doi.org/10.1016/j.jaci.2014.11.034. Tapia Granados, José A. and Diez Roux, Ana V. 'Life and death during the Great Depression'. https://doi.org/10.1073%2Fpnas.0904491106.

Thaiss, Christoph A. et al. 'Persistent microbiome alterations modulate the rate of post-dieting weight regain'. https://doi.org/10.1038/nature20796.

The Global Asthma Network. 'The global asthma report 2018'. http://globalasthmareport.org/resources/Global_Asthma_Report_2018.pdf.

Thorburn, Alison N. and Hansbro, Philip M. 'Harnessing Regulatory T cells to suppress asthma'. https://doi.org/10.1165%2Frcmb.2009-0342TR

Thorburn, Alison N., Macia, Laurence and Mackay, Charles. 'Diet, metabolites, and "western-lifestyle" inflammatory diseases'. https://doi.org/10.1016/j.immuni.2014.05.014.

Threapleton, Diane E. et al. 'Dietary fibre intake and risk of cardiovascular disease: Systematic review and meta-analysis'. https://doi.org/10.113 6/bmj.f6879.

Thursby, Elizabeth and Juge, Nathalie. 'Introduction to the human gut microbiota'. https://doi.org/10.1042/bcj20160510.

Turnbaugh, Peter J. et al. 'An obesity-associated gut microbiome with increased capacity for energy harvest'. https://doi.org/10.1038/nature05 414.

Turroni, Silvia et al. 'Temporal dynamics of the gut microbiota in people sharing a confined environment, a 520-day ground-based space simulation, MARS500'. https://doi.org/10.1186/s4 0168-017-0256-8.

Uebanso, Takashi et al. 'Functional roles of B-vitamins in the gut and gut microbiome'. https://doi.org/10.1002/mnfr.202000426.

Valadao, Priscila Aparecida Costa et al. 'Inflammation in Huntington's disease: A few new twists on an old tale'. https://www.sciencedirect .com/science/article/abs/pii/S0165572820305191.

Vaiserman, Alexander M., Koliada, Alexander K., Marotta, F. 'Gut microbiota: A player in aging and a target for anti-aging intervention'. https://doi.org/10.1016/j.arr.2017.01.001.

Vatic, Mirela, von Haehling, Stephan and Ebner, Nicole. 'Inflammatory biomarkers of frailty'. https://doi.org/10.1016/j.exger.2020.110858.

Vaughan, Annalicia et al. 'COPD and the gut-lung axis: the therapeutic potential of fibre'. https://doi.org/10.21037/jtd.2019.10.40.

Venegas, Daniela Parada et al. 'Short Chain Fatty Acids (SCFAs)-mediated gut epithelial and immune regulation and its relevance for inflammatory bowel diseases'. https://doi.org/10.3389/fimmu.2019.00277.

Verstraelen, Hans et al. 'Characterisation of the human uterine microbiome in non-pregnant women through deep sequencing of the V1-2 region of the 16S rRNA gene'. https://doi.org/10.7717/peerj.1602.

Wahnschaffe, Ulrich et al. 'Predictors of clinical response to gluten-free diet in patients diagnosed with diarrhea-predominant irritable bowel syndrome'. https://doi.org/10.1016/j.cgh.2007.03.021.

Wan, Yi et al. 'Effects of dietary fat on gut microbiota and faecal metabolites, and their relationship with cardiometabolic risk factors: a 6-month randomised controlled-feeding trial'. ht tps://gut.bmj.com/content/68/8/1417.

Watson, Henry et al. 'A randomised trial of the effect of omega-3 polyunsaturated fatty acid supplements on the human intestinal microbiota'. https://doi.org/10.1136/gutjnl-2017-314968.

Wells, David Ames. Recent Economic Changes: and their effect on the production and distribution of wealth and the well-being of society. University of California Libraries (1889).

Whittlesey, Derwent. 'Fixation of shifting cultivation'. https://doi.org/10.2307/140329.

Whittlesey, Derwent. 'Major agricultural regions of the earth'. https://doi.org/10.2307/2569535.

Wilck, Nicola et al. 'Salt-responsive gut commensal modulates T H 17 axis and disease'. https://doi.org/10.1038/nature24628.

Well+Good Editors. '5 ways to support brain health, according to a neuroscientist'. https://w

ww.wellandgood.com/brain-healthindicators-neuri
va/.

Westman, Walter E.'Measuring the inertia and resilience of Ecosystems'. https://doi.org/10.2307 /1307321.

Wexler, Hannah M. 'Bacteroides: The good, the bad, and the nitty-gritty'. https://doi.org/10.1128 /cmr.00008-07.

Wolters, Maike et al. 'Dietary fat, the gut microbiota, and metabolic health – A systematic review conducted within the MyNewGut project'. https://doi.org/10.1016/j.clnu.2018.12.024.

Wood, Lisa G. 'Diet, obesity, and asthma'. https ://doi.org/10.1513/annalsats.201702-124aw.

Wood, Lisa et al. 'Lycopene-rich treatments modify noneosinophilic airway inflammation in asthma: proof of concept'. https://pubmed.ncbi.n lm. nih.gov/18324527/.

Wood, Lisa et al. 'Manipulating antioxidant intake in asthma: a randomized controlled trial'. https: //doi.org/10.3945/ajcn.111.032623.

Wood, Lisa G., Garg, Manohar L. and Gibson, Peter G. 'A high-fat challenge increases airway inflammation and impairs bronchodilator recovery in asthma'. https://doi.org/10.1016/j.jaci.2011.01.036.

World Health Organization ('WHO'). 'Cancer'. https://www.who.int/newsroom/fact-sheets/detail/cancer.

World Health Organization ('WHO'). 'Chronic obstructive pulmonary disease (COPD)'. https://www.who.int/news-room/fact-sheets/detail/chronic-obstructive-pulmonary-disease-(copd).

World Health Organization ('WHO'). 'Global Health Estimates 2020: Deaths by cause, age, sex, by country and by region, 2000-2019'. https://www.who.int/data/gho/data/themes/mortality-and-globalhealth-estimates/ghe-leading-causes-of-death.

World Health Organization ('WHO'). 'Obesity and overweight'. https://www.who.int/en/news-room/fact-sheets/detail/obesity-andoverweight.

Wu, Gary D. 'Linking long-term dietary patterns with gut microbial enterotypes'. https://doi.org/10.1126/science.1208344.

Yang, H.S. and Eun, J.B. 'Fermentation and sensory characteristics of korean traditional fermented liquor (makgeolli) added with citron (citrus junos SIEB ex TANAKA) juice'. http://www.koreascience.or.kr/article/ArticleFullRecord.jsp?cn=SPGHB5_2011_v43n4_438.

Yates, Paul Lamartine. Food, land and manpower in Western Europe. St. Martin's Press (1960).

Yates, Paul Lamartine. Food production in Western Europe: An economic survey of agriculture in six countries. Longman (1940).

Zechner, Ellen L. 'Inflammatory disease caused by intestinal pathobionts'. https://doi.org/10.1016/j.mib.2017.01.011.

Zeevi, David et al. 'Personalized nutrition by prediction of glycemic responses'. https://doi.org/10.1016/j.cell.2015.11.001.

Zhang, Zhengxiao et al. 'Impact of fecal microbiota transplantation on obesity and metabolic syndrome: A systematic review'. https://doi.org/10.3390/nu11102291.

Zhen, Shihan. 'Dietary pattern is associated with obesity in Chinese children and adolescents: Data from China Health and Nutrition Survey (CHNS)'. https://doi.org/10.1186/s12937-018-0372-8.

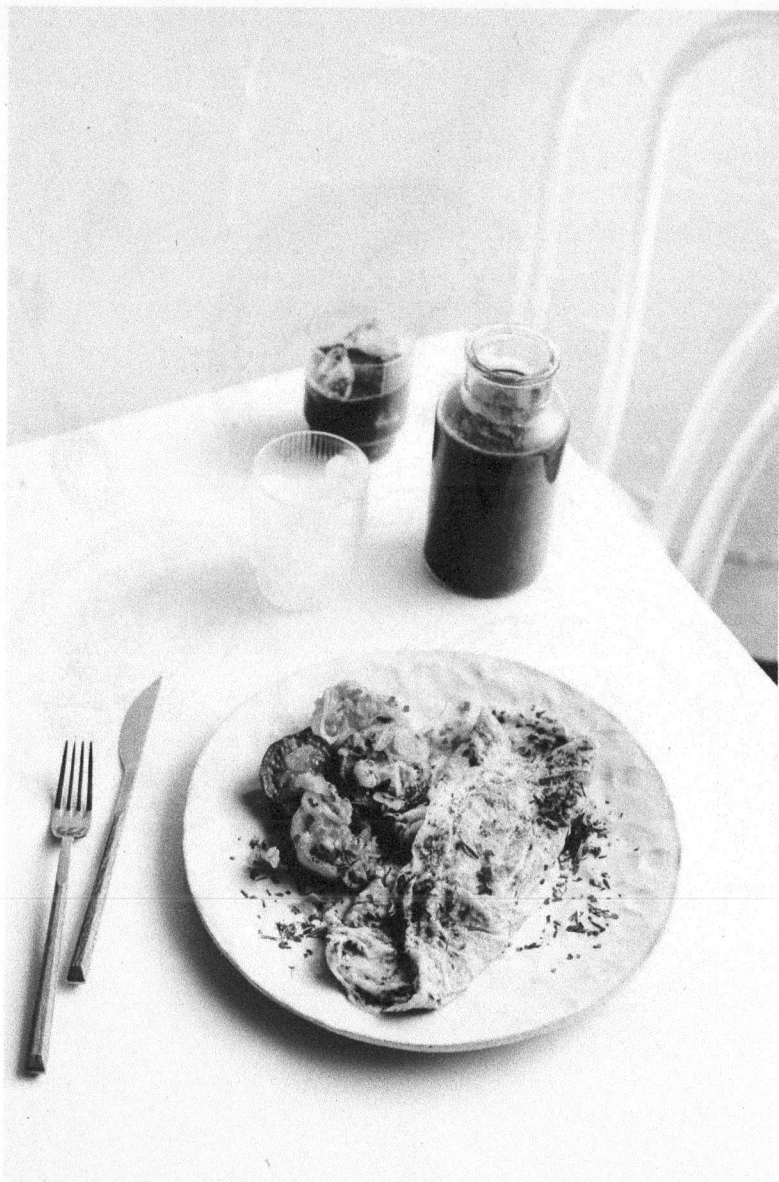

Green goddess breakfast smoothie with goat's milk yoghurt
(top) Herb omelettes with fried tomatoes (bottom)

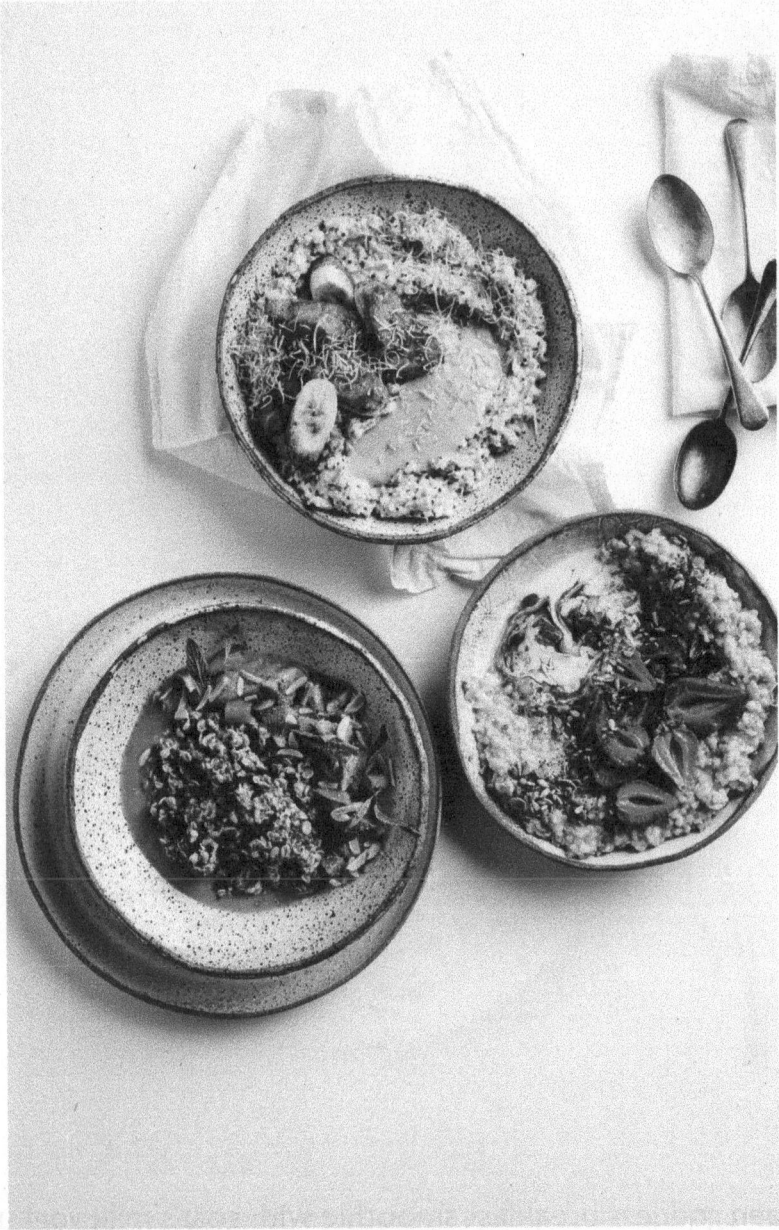

(clockwise from top) Coconut & tahini breakfast porridge with spiced banana Brown rice & buckwheat porridge with roasted strawberries & mixed seed sprinkle Overnight oats with papaya & kiwifruit

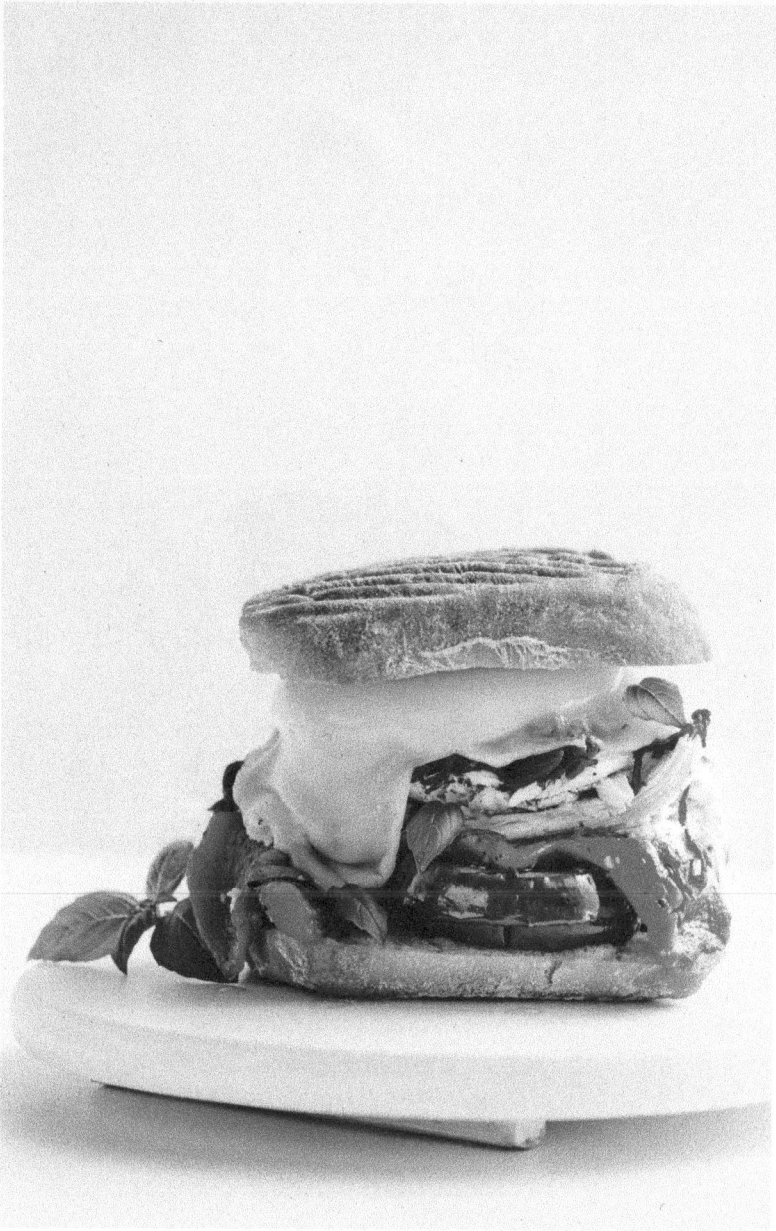

Roast chicken, sauerkraut & provolone pan bagnat

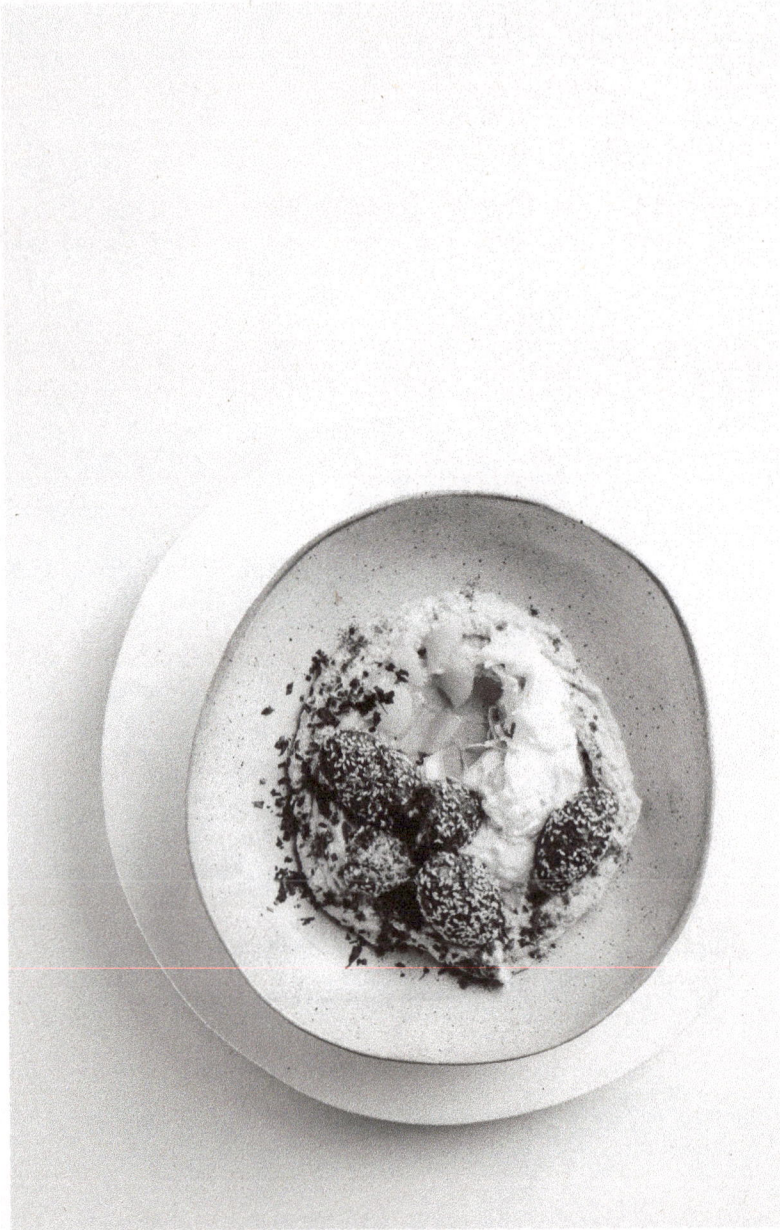

Parsley, dill & broad bean falafels with mint-garlic yoghurt

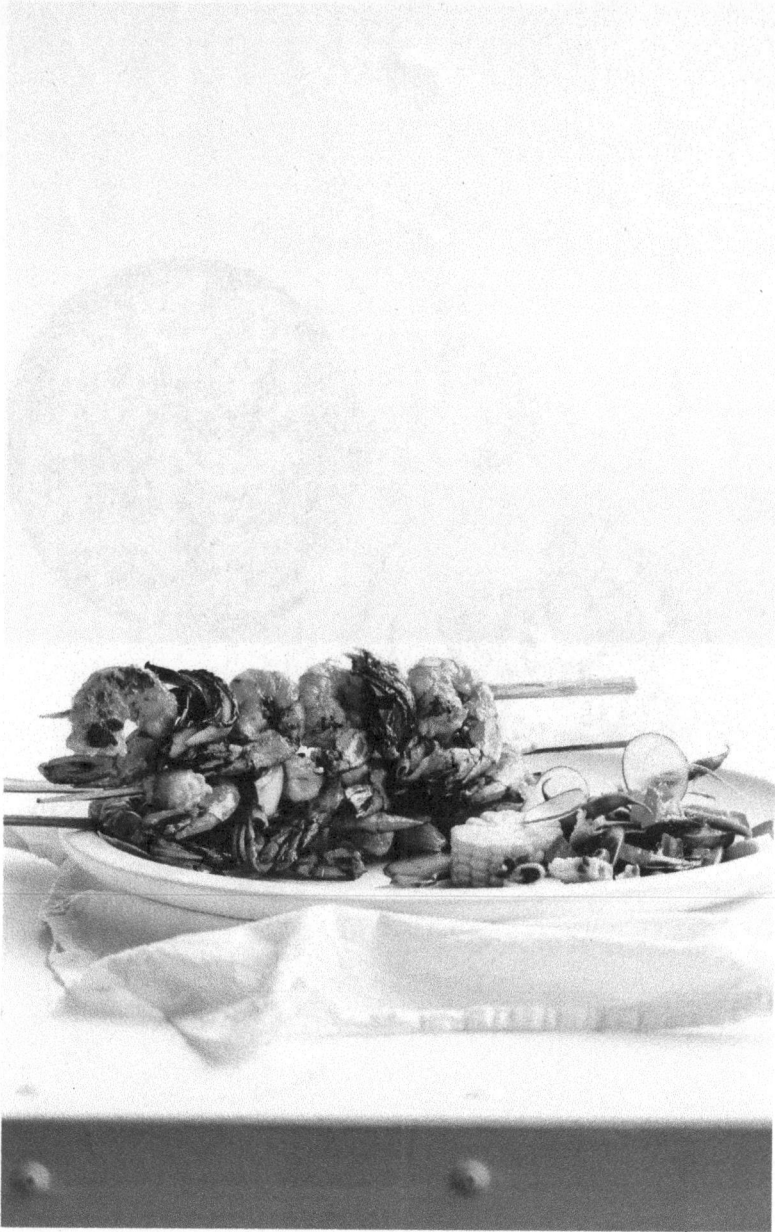

Prawn & onion kebabs with grilled corn & bean salad

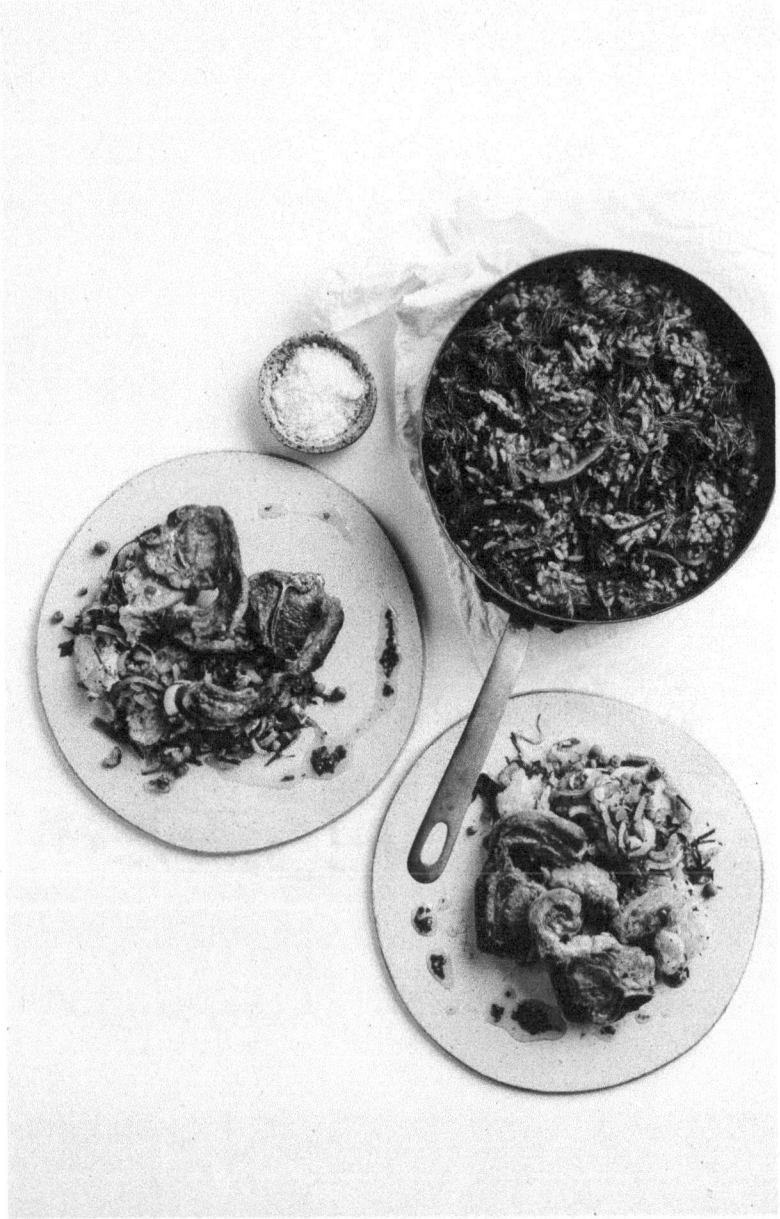

Roasted mushroom risotto (top right) Grass-fed lamb loin chops with whole-wheat kimchi dumplings in pea & garlic hash (bottom left and right)

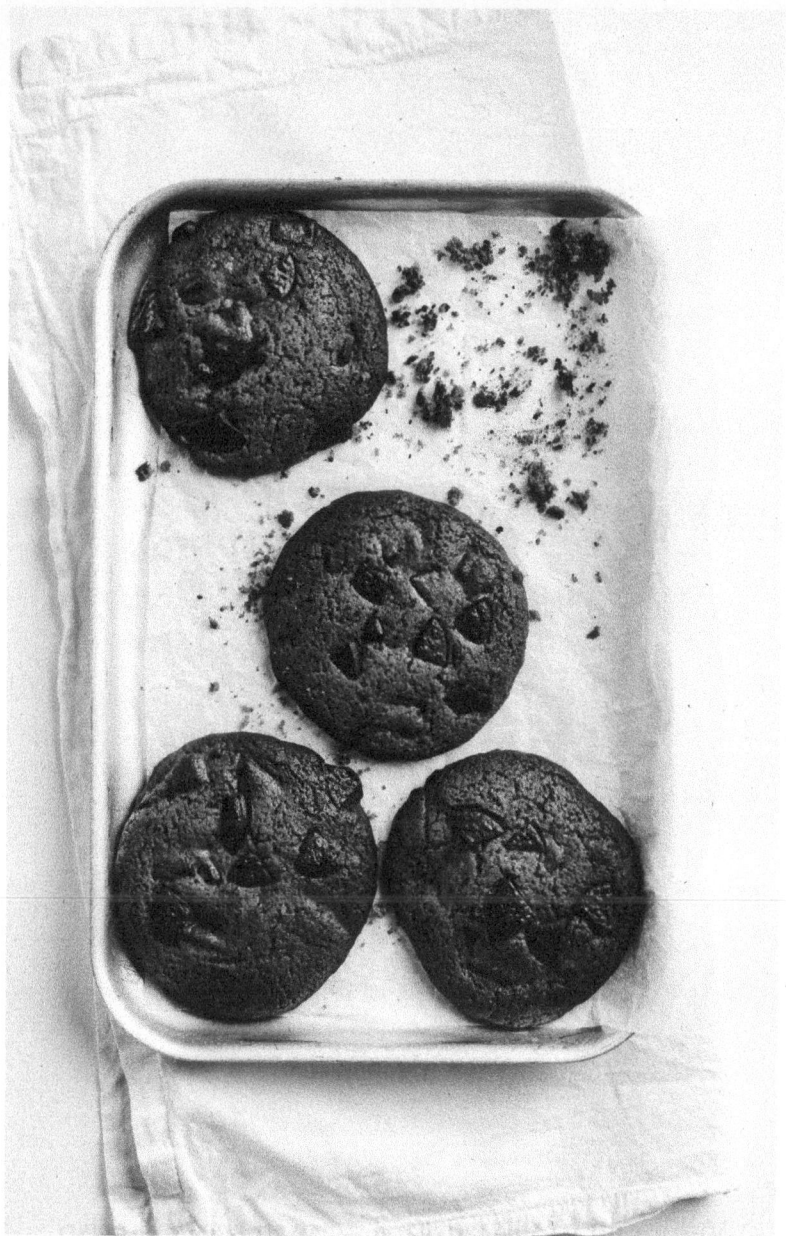

Easy olive oil chocolate-chunk cookies

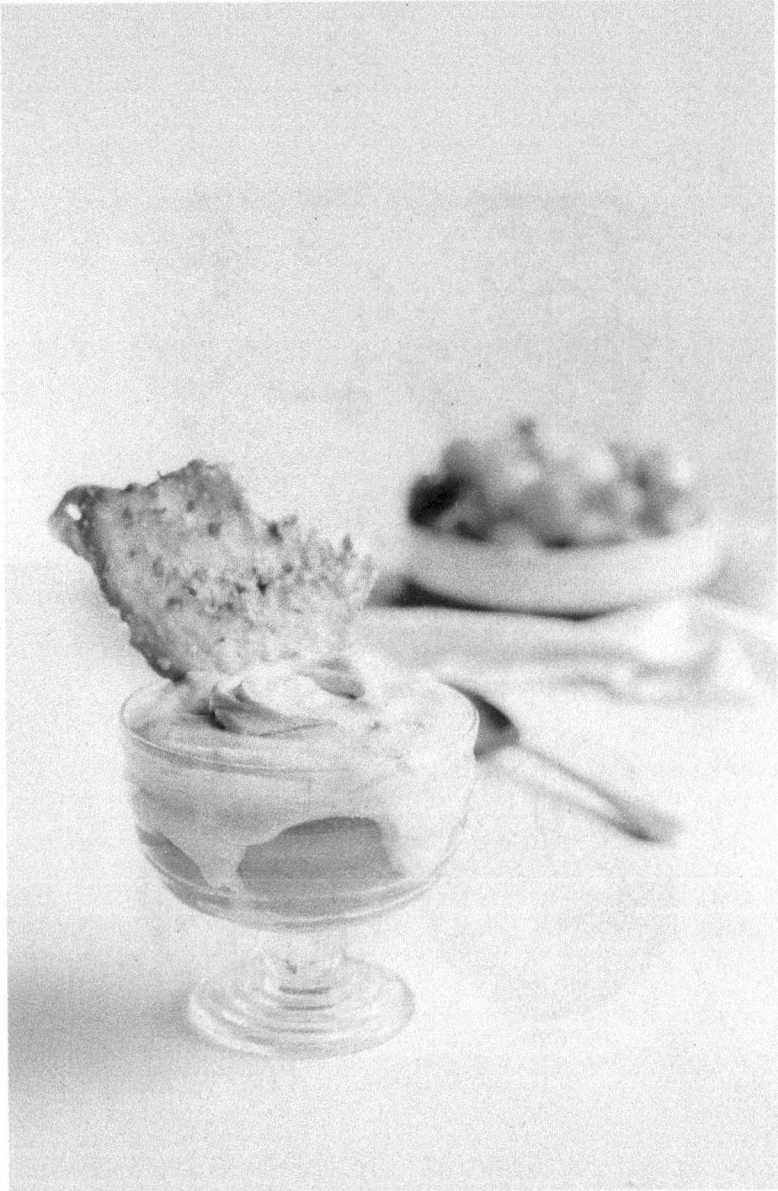

Whipped vanilla custard with apricots & crisp
parmesan-walnut wafers

Back Cover Material

At last, a book that shows you how to reverse the negative effects of inflammation, so you look and feel younger and live longer, happier and healthier.

For over four decades, world-leading independent medical research organisation the Centenary Institute has been producing breakthroughs in our biggest health challenges. Out of their mission to make people's lives better comes *The Good Gut Anti-Inflammatory Diet.*

- Understand inflammation, a fundamental cause of many life-altering diseases, and the various factors causing it
- Learn how balancing your gut with the right food choices can help manage inflammation and change your life
- Enjoy 50 versatile, delicious recipes from Aussie author and chef Fast Ed Halmagyi
- Benefit from nutrition tips and recipes from Dr Clare Bailey

Refocus on your health and energy, prevent sickness and reset yourself one delicious meal at a time.

A

acetate, *62, 72, 125*

adenosine triphosphate (ATP), *79*

ADHD, *145*

ageing,
  delaying, *36*
  hallmarks of, *35, 36*
  inflammation and, *34, 35, 36, 37, 38, 40*
  process of, *34, 35*

agriculture, rise of, *92, 93, 104*

Akkermansia bacteria, *37, 78, 83, 84*

alcohol, *127, 149, 150*

Alistipes, *76, 147*

allergic conditions, *4, 8, 50, 51, 57, 65, 68, 106, 119*
  rates of, *91*

Alzheimer's disease, *11, 13, 14, 34, 38, 40, 121*

amino acids, *70, 72, 83, 100, 150, 152*

animal-based foods, *83, 141, 143*

animal products, *155*

anthocyanins, *140*

antibiotics, *31, 44, 49, 51, 65, 71, 87, 100, 124, 143*

antioxidants, *71, 100, 131, 133, 134, 140, 150, 152*
  asthma and, *108*

anxiety, *119*

arthritis, *2, 8, 34, 35, 38, 57*
  rates of, *91*

artificial sweeteners, *149*

Asian diets, *93, 94*

asthma, *2, 4, 5, 8, 37, 44, 51, 57, 58, 63, 65, 68, 76, 83, 117*
  antioxidants an, *108*
  fat intake and, *107*
  fibre and, *108*
  healthy eating, *109*
  obesity and, *106, 107*
  rates of, *91*
  Western diets and, *104, 106, 107, 108, 109*

autoimmune conditions, *8, 11, 40, 50, 57, 147*

B

B vitamins, *80, 81, 102, 127, 150*

bacteria,
    dangerous, *58*
    number of, in gut, *70*
    nutritional needs, *70*
    symbiotic, *57, 58, 62, 65*

bacterial load, *65, 83*

Bacteroides, *76, 78, 80, 84, 136, 147*

Bacteroidetes, *50, 81*

beer, *150*

Bifidobacteria, *21, 59, 78, 154*

Bilophila, *78, 84*

blood glucose, *75, 125*

blood pressure, *11, 58*

Blue Zones', *130*

brain injury, traumatic, *11, 14*

breast cancer, *20, 59, 145*

butyrate, *61, 62, 72, 125, 152*

C

calorie restriction, *85*

cancers, *2, 18, 19, 20, 34, 35, 38, 40, 50*
    symptoms, *19*

carbohydrates, *70, 83, 84, 147*

cardiovascular diseases, *2, 11, 34, 40, 58, 59, 63, 68, 76, 84, 140, 141*

carotenoids, *109, 131*

Centenary Institute, *20, 67*

cholesterol, *11, 113, 145, 146, 150*

chronic diseases, *2, 20*
    age-related, *34, 40*
    diet and, *75, 76, 92, 100, 114, 154*
    fibre and, *137*
    inflammation and, *2, 3, 4, 5, 8, 11, 13, 14, 15, 17, 18, 19, 20, 21, 23, 75, 85*
    lifestyle-related, *68*
    maladaptive state, as, *75*
    preventing and treating, *103*
    rate of, *102, 103*
    Western diet and, *114*

chronic obstructive pulmonary disease (COPD), *2, 5, 34, 35, 38, 40, 50, 63, 91, 119, 125*

cider vinegar, *155, 274*

climate change, *127*

coeliac disease, *113*

colon cancer, *19, 53, 125, 137, 143*

COVID-19, *2, 4, 5*

Crohn's disease, *8, 119, 125*

cytomegalovirus (CMV), *36, 37*

D

dementia, *11, 14, 34, 35*

depression, *119, 145*

diabetes, *18, 59, 68, 112, 113, 117, 125, 130, 131, 137, 140, 141*

diarrhea, *23, 53, 71, 72*

diet,
    balanced, *150*
    changing, *30, 37, 127*
    disease and, *44, 75, 92, 100, 114, 154*
    diverse, *154*
    dysbiosis and, *75, 76*
    fibre-rich, *32*
    good, *68*
    gut friendly, *40*
    health and, *113*
    healthy, *109*
    high-fat, *37, 76, 83*
    high-protein, *84*
    holistic approach, *127*
    improving, *63*
    microbiome's composition and, *66, 68, 71, 72, 74, 75, 78, 133*
    overall health an, *72*
    pattern of food intake, as, *75*
    poor, *78, 85, 92*
    quality of, *154*
    through the ages, *92*
    well-balanced, *67*
    'whole of diet' approach, *103*

dietary fibre, *47, 58, 59, 61, 72, 76, 85, 100, 134, 135, 136, 137, 152*
    asthma and, *108, 109*
    chronic diseases and, *137*
    lung health and, *108*
    nutrition tip, *59*

soluble or insoluble, 108, 136, 139

sources of, 137

dietary guidelines, 129, 130

disease,

causes and effects, 88

chronic,

see chronic diseases,

diet and, 44, 75, 92, 100, 114, 154

inflammatory, 117

DNA, 111, 112

ageing and, 35

bacterial, 48

mutations, 18

drug-based treatments, 117

dysbiosis, 63, 65, 66

diet and, 75, 76

E

eating,

good health, for, 103

healthy eating, 150

mindful, 88

moderate intake, 155

overeating, 155

what we should eat, 150

emphysema, 5, 35, 40, 91, 116, 119

endotoxins, 56, 136

Enterococcus, 84

epigenetics, 111, 112

Escherichia coli, 53, 80, 84

Europe, Northwest, 96, 97, 98

exercise, 119, 120, 123, 155

resistance, 123

F

factory farming, 143

faecal transfers, 111, 124, 125

Faecalibacterium, 58, 61, 76, 84, 136

fats, 70, 83, 102, 147

asthma and fat intake, 107

dietary fats, 144

good and bad, 144

fermented foods, 135, 155

fibre,

see dietary fibre,

Firmicutes, 50, 81

flavonoids, 109

flavonols, *139*
folate, *127*
food,
  availability, *112*
  discretionary, *106, 155*
  diversity, *89*
  fermented, *135*
  fresh, *150*
  high rotation foods, *152*
  industrialisation, *100*
  key concepts, *154, 155*
  preservation, *98*
  processed, *91*
  processing, stages of, *98*
  quality of, *129*
  real, *78, 144*
  scarcity and abundance, *74*
  unprocessed, *113, 150*
  whole grain, *141*
food additives, *149*
food allergies, *8, 65, 119*
'free radicals', *109, 133, 140*
fruits, *155*

G
genetics, *111, 112*

germ-free studies, *46, 47, 49*
gluten, *147*
glycolysis, *79, 80*
GPR receptors, *62*
gut,
  immune system and, *32*
  purpose, *55*
gut microbiome, *42, 43, 44, 46, 47, 48, 49, 50, 51, 53*
  ageing and, *37*
  birth, at, *47*
  changing, *53*
  diet and disease, *44*
  diet and,
    see diet,
  diversity in, *53, 67, 154*
  dynamic and distinct, *53*
  healthy, *88*
  immune system and, *55, 56, 57, 58, 133*
  inflammation and, *37, 55, 56, 57, 58, 59, 61, 62, 63, 65, 66, 67*
  microbiome-based therapies, *124*
  modifying, *67*

out-of-balance, 63
sequencing, 125
studying, 47, 48, 49

H
hay fever, 8, 65, 119
healthy ingredients, 155
heart attack, 8, 11, 40
heart disease, 2, 5, 11, 35, 91, 102, 112, 113, 119, 125, 130, 131, 133, 137, 141, 144, 150
hepatitis, 18, 19
Huntington's disease, 11, 14

I
immune system, 32, 36, 38, 44, 46, 50, 51, 116
adaptive immunity, 28, 29
gut and, 32
innate, 24, 25
microbes and, 72
microbiome and, 55, 56, 57, 58, 133
sleep and, 121
immune, tolerance, 57, 58, 65
'immunobiography', 36
indole compounds, 58, 80

infertility, 15
'inflammageing', 34
disease, and, 38
rise of, 38
inflammation, 20, 23, 24, 25, 26, 28, 29, 30, 31, 32, 116
acute, signs of, 26
ageing and, 34, 35, 36, 37, 38, 40
cancer and, 18
chronic, 28, 29, 30
chronic diseases, 2, 3, 4, 5, 8, 11, 13, 14, 15, 17, 18, 19, 20, 21, 85
chronic intestinal, 75
excess macronutrients and, 81
gut microbiome influencing, 37, 55, 56, 57, 58, 59, 61, 62, 63, 65, 66, 67
intestinal, 75
lifestyle approaches to minimising, 119
minimising, 116, 117, 119, 120, 121, 123, 124, 125, 127
modern triggers, 30, 31, 32
natural immune system defence, 23

inflammatory bowel disease, *2, 8, 58, 63, 124, 125, 143*

  rates of, *91*

inflammatory processes, *2, 3, 56*

influenza, *2, 4, 5, 23, 119*

intermittent fasting, *85, 87*

intestinal inflammation, *75*

iron, *80, 113, 154*

K

kidney disease, *2, 8, 17, 119, 143, 150*

kimchi, *135, 155*

L

Lactobacillus, *59, 78, 134, 136*

lactose intolerance, *113*

leaky gut, *62, 81, 83, 120, 125, 136, 147*

life expectancy, *2, 4, 5, 23, 34, 112, 119*

  Japan, in, *130*

  poor diet and lifestyle, *92*

lifestyle,

  changing, *30*

  chronic diseases and, *68*

  healthy, *40, 67, 109*

  holistic approach, *127*

  improving, *63*

  inflammation, minimising, *119*

  poor, *92*

liver disease, *2, 17, 18, 125*

lung cancer, *20*

lupus, *8*

M

macronutrients, *76*

  distribution, *85*

  excess, *81*

meal planner, *158*

meat,

  animal-based foods, *83, 141, 143*

  grass-fed and grain-fed, *143*

Mediterranean diet, *94, 96, 103, 131, 133, 146, 155*

meningitis, *11, 14, 119*

mental illnesses, *63*

metabolites, *55, 56, 58, 63, 65, 67, 70, 71, 76, 125, 136*

  effects, *125*

microbes,
  by-products from, 72
  immune system and, 72
  sources of carbon and energy, 72
microbiome,
  see gut microbiome,
microbiota, 42, 49, 50, 51, 53, 56, 88, 124, 130, 144, 147, 149
micronutrients, 76, 78
mindful eating, 88
mitochondria, 79, 80
monounsaturated fatty acids, 144, 146
multiple sclerosis, 8, 14, 57, 62, 116

N
neurological conditions, 2, 11, 117
nutrition,
  importance of, 129
  tips, 59, 78, 87, 88, 113, 121, 123, 135, 140, 146, 274
  understanding, 103

O
obesity, 18, 19, 111, 125, 130, 131
  asthma and, 106, 107
  genetics, 111
  predicting, 49
  rates of, 91, 92, 106, 107
Okinawan diet, 103, 130, 131, 133, 155
olive oil, 94, 96, 100, 131, 134, 140, 145, 146, 155, 274
Omega-3 fatty acids, 145, 146, 147, 152, 154
Omega-6 unsaturated fats, 144
oxidative phosphorylation, 79

P
Parkinson's disease, 11, 13, 14
pathogens, 56, 57, 67, 85
peanut allergy, 134
periodontitis, 37
phytochemicals, 139, 140
plant-based foods, 78, 83, 84, 93, 103, 109, 130, 131, 133, 136, 140, 152, 155
  phytochemicals, 139

pneumonia, *2, 4, 5, 23, 119*
polyphenols, *139, 140*
polyunsaturated fatty
acids, *37, 144, 145, 146, 147*
prebiotics, *134, 135*
Prevotella, *58, 59, 136*
probiotics, *21, 125, 134, 135*
  supplements, *124*
processed foods, *58, 67,*
91, 103, 130, 131, 150, 154
propionate, *61, 62, 72*
protein, *83, 141*
Proteobacteria, *70, 80*
psoriasis, *8, 119, 134, 135*

R
reductionism, *102, 103*
Reproductive tract
conditions, *15*
respiratory diseases, *4,*
141
Ruminococcus, *84*

S
salt intake, excessive, *80*
saturated fatty acids, *37,*
76, 83, 107, 144, 145
seaweed, *146*
seeds and nuts, *155*
senescent cells, *35, 38*

sexually transmitted
infections, *15*
short-chain fatty acids
(SCFAs), *21, 57, 58, 61, 62,*
72, 108, 111, 146, 147
  inflammation,
  preventing, *62*
sleep, *119, 121*
  hygiene, *121*
smoking, *5, 8, 11, 19, 20, 98,*
119
  quitting, *127*
starch, resistant, *61, 136*
  sources of, *139*
Streptococcus, *84*
stress, *119, 120, 121*
stressors, *120*
stroke, *11, 13, 40, 91, 119,*
131
sugar, excessive, *85*
symbiotic relationship,
66
systemic inflammation,
3, 20

T
T-cells, *57, 80*
time restricted eating, *87*
trans fats, *145*

tuberculosis, *3, 5, 117, 119*
type 1 diabetes, *8, 40, 57, 113*
type 2 diabetes, *121*

U
ulcerative colitis, *8, 125*

V
vasculitis, *8, 119*
Verrucomicrobia, *80*
vitamins,
  B vitamins, *80, 81, 102, 127, 150*
  discovery of, *102*
  vitamin C, *71, 72, 78, 102, 108*
  vitamin E, *71, 72, 78, 109*

W
walking, *121*
Western diet, *100, 102, 113, 114*
  asthma and, *104, 106, 107, 108, 109*
  chronic disease, *114*
  rise of, *91*
whole grain foods, *141, 155*

'whole of diet' approach, *103*
wine, *150*